# The Physician's
# Book of Lists

# THE PHYSICIAN'S BOOK OF LISTS

## David M. Margulies, M.D.

Columbia Presbyterian Medical Center
New York, New York

## and

## Malcolm S. Thaler, M.D.

New England Deaconess Hospital
Boston, Massachusetts

Churchill Livingstone 1983
New York, Edinburgh, London, Melbourne

Distributed in the United Kingdom by Churchill Livingstone,
Robert Stevenson House, 1–3 Baxter's Place, Leith Walk,
Edinburgh EH1 3AF and associated companies, branches
and representatives throughout the world.

First published 1983
Printed in U.S.A.

ISBN 0-443-08178-6
9  8  7  6  5  4  3


Library of Congress Cataloging in Publication Data

Margulies, David.
  The physician's book of lists.
  1. Diagnosis—Outlines, syllabi, etc.   I. Thaler,
Malcolm S.  II. Title.  [DNLM: 1. Diagnosis.
2. Medicine.  WB 141 M331p]
RC71.3.M28 1983     616.07'5              82-19883
ISBN 0-443-08178-6


Manufactured in the United States of America

# Preface

Everyone makes lists—it has, in recent years, even become something of a national pastime—but few do so with the fervor and sheer profusion as physicians. Whether hastily scribbled on a blackboard during rounds or meticulously copied into a little black book and stuffed into one's jacket pocket, lists comprise a fundamental part of one's clinical armamentarium: differential diagnoses, signs and symptoms, drug interactions and side effects, diagnostic protocols, etiologic considerations. Their number is limitless, a function of the vast wealth of clinical information and the urgent necessity to organize it all into focused, functional portions.

Lists are efficient and effective. However, they contain little clinical judgment. A list merely provides terse data to be processed within the framework of clinical judgment. One must bring one's education and experience *to* a list. Only then can the dangers of oversimplification and missed subtleties be avoided. Lists jog the memory, organize one's thoughts, clarify one's approach. They do not in themselves educate or instill clinical acumen. Lists are merely the tersest condensation of ideas which are developed, defended, and given context elsewhere.

Nevertheless, used with care, lists make better, more confident physicians of us all. We have tried here to select those lists that have proven most useful for us and for many other active clinicians. This book is hardly exhaustive. It could easily have been ten times as large and the paring down to portable size was often a difficult process. We hope the end result addresses a wide sampling of the key questions encountered in the everyday practice of medicine. The emphasis is clearly on diagnosis and approach. Therapeutics are represented only sporadically, largely because of the large number of outstanding therapeutic manuals already available.

We view this book as an on-going project, and hope that you will send us some of your favorite lists for possible inclusion in future editions. Please send them to:

David M. Margulies, M.D. and Malcolm S. Thaler, M.D.
c/o Churchill Livingstone Inc.
1560 Broadway
New York, New York 10036

We wish to give special thanks to Mr. Lewis Reines, who conceived this project and whose warm humor, gentle guidance, and deft prodding made this book a reality. Acknowledgements plunge too readily into the sentimental, but to Lew we simply cannot overstate our appreciation and feelings of friendship. We would also like to express our deepest gratitude to our families and friends for their constant support, and especially to Else Smedemark and Nancy Klinghoffer, whose love and encouragement are the best medicine of all.

                                                    M.T.
                                                    D.M.

# Contents

## Section 2. Pulmonary Disease                    53

## Section 3. Endocrinology 87

# Section 6. Fluids and Electrolytes 171

# Section 7. Nephrology 191

# Section 8. Gastroenterology 211

## Section 9. Neurology                                    255

## Section 10. Miscellaneous Lists      281

# Section

# 1

# Cardiology

## IMPORTANT CAUSES OF SHOCK

1. Cardiogenic
   a. Myocardial infarction (15% of acute MIs)
   b. Valvular disease (especially acute mitral regurgitation)
   c. Congestive failure
   d. Arrhythmias (especially ventricular tachycardia)
   e. Obstructive disease (especially pulmonary embolism, pneumo-thorax and cardiac tamponade)
   f. Toxic: (1) endogenous — circulating vasoactive toxins, such as myocardial depressant factors; and (2) exogenous—cardiotoxic drug overdoses, e.g., tricylic antidepressants
2. Hypovolemic
   a. Hemorrhage
   b. Burns
   c. Trauma
   d. Ruptured aneurysm
   e. Anaphylaxis
   f. Disseminated intravascular coagulation (DIC)
   g. Pancreatitis (due to both volume loss and the release of myo-cardial depressant factors)
   h. Peritonitis
3. Septic (generally gram negative sepsis)
4. Other
   a. Addison's disease
   b. Neurogenic (spinal cord injuries, narcotic/barbiturate over-dose)

## HYPODYNAMIC VS. HYPERDYNAMIC SHOCK

|  | *Hypodynamic Shock* | *Hyperdynamic Shock* |
| --- | --- | --- |
| *Major causes* | Cardiogenic, hypovolemic | Septic |
| Patient's skin | Cool, clammy | Warm, flushed |
| Blood pressure | Decreased | Decreased |
| Pulse | Increased | Increased |
| Cardiac output | Decreased | Increased early, decreased later |
| AV O$_2$ difference | Increased | Decreased early, increased later |
| Total peripheral resistance | Increased | Decreased early, increased later |
| Pulmonary capillary wedge pressure | Increased in cardiogenic shock Decreased in hypovolemic shock | Decreased |
| Central venous pressure | Increased in cardiogenic shock Decreased in hypovolemic shock | Decreased |
| Lactate levels | Increased | Increased |

## MANAGEMENT OF THE PATIENT IN SHOCK:
### Essential Measurements

1. Vital signs: blood pressure, pulse, temperature, respiratory rate
2. Assessment of mental status, adequacy of distal perfusion
3. Serum electrolytes, glucose, creatinine, BUN
4. Urine output and osmolality; urinary sodium concentration
5. Hemoglobin, hematocrit, white blood cell and platelet counts
6. Arterial blood gases
7. Central venous pressure (or, preferably, pulmonary capillary wedge pressure)
8. ECG and chest x-ray
9. In appropriate patients:
   a. blood cultures
   b. fibrin, fibrin split products, fibrinogen and complement levels
10. Record all fluid input and output and time and amount of all drugs

### Specific Therapeutic Measures

1. Maintain intravascular volume with goal of CVP 10–12 mm Hg; PCW 18–20 mm Hg. Give whole blood, saline, or colloids as appropriate
2. Correct hypoxemia to $Po_2$ > 60 mm Hg. Use increasing $FIO_2$ values; intubate and use pressure cycled respirator technique if needed
3. Correct acidosis
4. If hypotension persists, use pressors. In general, isoproterenol (Isoprel) is used when generalized beta adrenergic effects are desired; dopamine (Inotropin) is used in low doses for maintaining renal perfusion, and in higher doses as a mixed alpha and beta agent; norepinephrine (Levophed) is used for its alpha effects and dobutamine (Dobutex) is used for cardiac inotropic beta stimulation.
5. Treat specific precipitants (CHF, sepsis, adrenal insufficiency, hemorrhage, etc.)

# THE AMERICAN HEART ASSOCIATION'S CLASSIFICATION OF PATIENTS WITH HEART DISEASE *

## Functional Classification

Class I: Patients with cardiac disease but without resulting limitation of physical activity. Ordinary physical activity does not cause undue fatigue, palpitation, dyspnea, or anginal pain.

Class II: Patients with cardiac disease resulting in slight limitation of physical activity. They are comfortable at rest. Ordinary physical activity results in fatigue, palpitation, dyspnea, or anginal pain.

Class III: Patients with cardiac disease resulting in marked limitation of physical activity. They are comfortable at rest. Less than ordinary activity causes fatigue, palpitation, dyspnea, or anginal pain.

Class IV: Patients with cardiac disease resulting in inability to carry on any physical activity without discomfort. Symptoms of cardiac insufficiency or of the anginal syndrome are present even at rest. If any physical activity is undertaken, discomfort is increased.

## Therapeutic Classification

Class A: Patients with a cardiac disease whose ordinary physical activity need not be restricted.

Class B: Patients with cardiac disease whose ordinary physical activity need not be restricted, but who should be advised against severe or competitive physical efforts.

Class C: Patients with cardiac disease whose ordinary physical activity should be moderately restricted, and whose more strenuous efforts should be discontinued.

Class D: Patients with cardiac disease whose ordinary physical activity should be markedly restricted.

Class E: Patients with cardiac disease who should be at complete rest, confined to bed or chair.

*Excerpted from Diseases of the Heart and Blood Vessels—Nomenclature and Criteria for Diagnosis, 6th edition, Boston, Little Brown and Company, copyright 1964 by the New York Heart Association, Inc. These classifications are not included in the 7th edition, revised 1973, nor in the 8th edition, revised 1979.

## IMPORTANT CAUSES OF CHEST PAIN

1. Myocardial pain
   a. Angina
      i. Dull, heavy, pressurelike pain
      ii. Substernal, may radiate to arms, shoulders, jaw, neck
      iii. Does not persist for more than a few minutes
      iv. Brought on by exertion, emotion, eating
      v. Relieved by nitroglycerin and rest
      vi. Associated symptoms may include anxiety, dyspnea, sweating, nausea, vomiting
      vii. Physical exam during an attack reveals tachycardia, an $S_4$ or $S_3$ gallop, a parodoxically split $S_2$; ECG reveals ST depression and T wave inversion
   b. Prinzmetal's (variant") angina
      i. Anginal pain at rest
      ii. Associated with ST elevation
   c. Acute myocardial infarction
      i. Pain identical to angina, but more prolonged and severe
2. Pericardial pain
   a. Pericarditis
      i. Sharp, stabbing pain
      ii. Substernal or parasternal, may radiate to neck or shoulders, rarely down arms
      iii. Intensity affected by respiration and position; typically most severe in left lateral decubitus position and relieved by sitting up and leaning forward
      iv. A friction rub may be heard on physical exam
3. Pleural and pulmonary pain
   a. Pleuritic pain
      i. Sharp pain, often rapid in onset
      ii. Usually localized to one side, frequently to a particular spot
      iii. Worsened by coughing and respiration
      iv. Often not relieved by changes in position
      v. Patient is sometimes tachypneic
      vi. Physical exam reveals patient to be splinting the affected side
   b. Pulmonary embolus
      i. Pain is typically pleuritic
      ii. Associated symptoms may include dyspnea, hemoptysis or syncope
      iii. Classical triad of pleuritic pain, dyspnea, and hemoptysis occurs in less than 30% of patients

      iv. A massive embolus may produce a dull, substernal pain resembling angina

  c. Pneumothorax

      i. Pain is pleuritic

      ii. Physical exam reveals hyperresonance, with decreased breath sounds

  d. Pulmonary hypertension

      i. Dull, aching pain similar to angina

      ii. Substernal

      iii. Pain is related to stress and exertion

      iv. Patient is frequently dyspneic

4. Costochondral pain

  a. Tietze's syndrome

      i. Dull, aching pain

      ii. Usually located over cartilage of ribs 2, 3, or 4

      iii. Exacerbated by chest movement, respiration, coughing

      iv. Relieved by anti-inflammatory medication

      v. Physical exam reveals tenderness over costochondral joints; pain can be elicited by applying pressure over affected areas

5. Aortic pain

  a. Aortic dissection

      i. Tearing pain, sudden in onset

      ii. Substernal, may radiate to back and abdomen

      iii. Pain is often most intense at onset

      iv. Physical exam frequently reveals peripheral pulse deficits

6. Gastrointestinal pain

  a. Esophagitis and esophageal spasm

      i. Deep, burning pain

      ii. May radiate to shoulder

      iii. Frequently follows meals

      iv. Often relieved by antacids or nitroglycerin

  b. Splenic flexure syndrome

      i. Feeling of pressure or fullness

      ii. Originates in upper abdomen and radiates to left chest, sometimes to left shoulder and arm

      iii. Relieved by defecation or expulsion of flatus

  c. Other gastrointestinal disorders in which pain may radiate to the chest

      i. Gastritis

      ii. Peptic ulcer disease

      iii. Pancreatitis

      iv. Biliary colic

## IMPORTANT CAUSES OF CHEST PAIN *(cont.)*

7. Intercostal neuritis
   a. Herpes zoster (shingles)
      i. Usually superficial tingling, but may be deep and burning
      ii. Felt in dermatome distribution
      iii. Physical exam may reveal dysesthesia and rash in same distribution
8. Other causes of chest pain
   a. Muscle strain: localized tenderness, related to movement
   b. Fractured ribs: localized point tenderness; pain may be severe and disabling
   c. Sickle cell crisis: diffuse gnawing pain that increases over several hours and affects the chest, but also the abdomen, arms, and joints

## THE JUGULAR AND CAROTID PULSES

### The Jugular Venous Pulse*

The normal jugular venous pulse, best viewed on the right side of the neck, consists of three waves.

1. The *A wave* is due to rebound from atrial systole. It is visible as a flicker just prior to the carotid pulse. It is followed by the *X descent*, representing atrial relaxation.
2. The *C wave* is due to bulging of the tricuspid valve upon closure. It coincides with the carotid pulse, but is rarely visible. When seen, the descent following it is called *X'*.
3. The *V wave* is due to atrial filling while the tricuspid valve is closed. It is visible as a prolonged wave just following the carotid pulse. It is followed by the *Y descent*, corresponding to the fall in venous pressure upon reopening of the tricuspid valve.

| *Abnormality in the JVP* | *Causes* |
|---|---|
| Elevated venous pressures | Cardiac tamponade, chronic constrictive pericarditis, right heart failure, hypervolemia, obstruction of the superior vena cava |
| Kussmaul's sign (inspiratory rise in JVP) | Chronic constrictive pericarditis |
| Large A waves | Tricuspid stenosis, pulmonic stenosis, right ventricular hypertrophy, septal hypertrophy |
| "Cannon" A waves | AV dissociation |
| Absent A waves | Atrial fibrillation |
| Large V waves | Tricuspid regurgitation |
| Prominent X descent | Cardiac tamponade |
| Prominent Y descent | Chronic constrictive pericarditis |

### The Carotid Pulse

| *Abnormality in the Carotid Pulse* | *Causes* |
|---|---|
| Wide pulse pressure | Aortic regurgitation, abnormal AV communication, thyrotoxicosis, fever, anemia, beriberi heart |
| Narrow pulse pressure | Aortic stenosis, tachycardia |

* The jugular venous pressure only measures pressures on the *right side* of the heart.

## THE JUGULAR AND CAROTID PULSES *(cont.)*

| *Abnormality in the Carotid Pulse* | *Causes* |
| --- | --- |
| Pulsus bisferiens (two systolic peaks) | Asymmetric septal hypertrophy (ASH), ventricular septal defect (VSD), aortic regurgitation |
| Pulsus tardus (plateau pulse) | Aortic stenosis |
| Pulsus alternans (pulse waves alternate in size) | Myocardial weakness |
| Pulsus paradoxus (inspiratory fall in arterial systolic pressure of >10 mm Hg) | Pericardial tamponade, obstructive pulmonary disease, myocardial disease |

## PALPITATIONS: DIFFERENTIAL DIAGNOSIS

Palpitations, the awareness, usually unpleasant, of one's heartbeat, can be caused by almost any disturbance in cardiac rhythm or rate. Ventricular tachycardia, however, usually does not cause palpitations. Some causes of palpitations are listed below:

1. Isolated palpitations
   a. Extrasystoles (atrial, junctional, or ventricular premature contractions)
2. Paroxysmal palpitations
   a. Paroxysmal supraventricular tachycardias
   b. Atrial flutter
   c. Atrial fibrillation
   d. Supraventricular tachycardias with constant ratio heart block
   e. Orthostatic hypotension
   f. Anxiety
   g. Pheochromocytoma
   h. Hypoglycemia
   i. Drugs and stimulants (e.g., caffeine, tobacco, amphetamines, amyl nitrate, aminophylline, sympathomimetics)
   j. Migraine
   k. Menopausal syndrome
3. Persistent palpitations
   a. States of high output and increased stroke volume
      i. Thyrotoxicosis
      ii. Anemia
      iii. Volume depletion
      iv. Fever
      v. Beriberi
      vi. Abnormal AV communication
      vii. Pregnancy
      viii. Aortic or mitral regurgitation
   b. Anxiety
   c. Bradycardia
   d. Mild exercise in patients who are in poor physical condition

## ELEVATED SERUM ENZYMES IN ACUTE MYOCARDIAL INFARCTION

| Enzyme | Earliest Rise | Peak | Normalizes | False Positives | Myocardial Isoenzyme | Comments |
|---|---|---|---|---|---|---|
| CK | 3–6 h | 12–24 h | 3–4 days | Skeletal muscle injury (e.g., from IM injection), pulmonary embolism, hypothyroidism, cerbrovascular disease | MB | Earliest indicator of infarction |
| SGOT | 6–12 h | 1–2 days | 3–4 days | Liver disease, renal disease, skeletal muscle injury, pulmonary embolism, cerebrovascular disease, use of oral contraceptives | — | Very high levels suggest acute hepatic injury from shock |
| LDH | 1–2 days | 2–6 days | 7–14 days | Liver disease, pulmonary embolism, neoplasms, anemias (esp. hemolytic and megaloblastic) | $LDH_1$ (also present in red blood cells) | Valuable on suspicion that an MI occurred several days earlier; $LDH_1$ > $LDH_2$ strongly suggests infarction |

## ACUTE MYOCARDIAL INFARCTION: COMPLICATIONS

| *Complication* | *Comments* |
| --- | --- |
| 1. Sudden death | Fifty percent of deaths from an acute MI occur within the first 2–3 h. |
| 2. Arrhythmias | Arrhythmias are the leading cause of death in acute MI; the most common arrhythmias are ventricular extrasystoles, followed by sinus tachycardia, ventricular tachycardia, and sinus bradycardia; nevertheless, virtually any arrhythmia can occur. |
| 3. Heart block | In patients with inferior MIs, heart block is generally transient; heart block in patients with anterior MIs may require a pacemaker. |
| 4. Congestive heart failure and cardiogenic shock | Congestive heart failure is common; cardiogenic shock may supervene when more than 40% of the left ventricle is destroyed. |
| 5. Ventricular rupture | Free wall rupture presents as electromechanical dissociation with blood in the pericardial sac; septal rupture presents with a new loud systolic murmur in the third or fourth intercostal space; both require emergency surgical repair. |
| 6. Pulmonary and systemic emboli | Patients with congestive failure, especially when complicated by atrial fibrillation, a large ventricular aneurysm or deep vein thrombosis should be anticoagulated. |
| 7. Mitral regurgitation | Usually not significant unless due to papillary muscle rupture, in which case shock may develop. Papillary rupture is most common with IMIs, usually occurs 2 to 7 days post MI, and requires valve replacement. |
| 8. Pericarditis | One third of patients develop a friction rub; tamponade is rare. |
| 9. Dressler's syndrome | One to five percent of patients develop a syndrome of pericarditis, pleuritis, myalgias, arthralgias, and fever several weeks to months following an acute MI. |

## TREATMENT OF CARDIAC ARRHYTHMIAS

### Supraventricular Arrhythmias

1. Atrial fibrillation
    a. If urgent, DC cardioversion
    b. Verapamil*
    c. Cardioversion can be attempted with digitalis followed by quinidine.
    d. If the patient is stable, digitalis or propranolol can be used to slow the ventricular rate
2. Atrial flutter: as above
3. Paroxysmal supraventricular tachycardia
    a. Vagal maneuvers (carotid sinus massage, Valsalva maneuver, diving reflex, etc.)
    b. Verapamil, digitalis, or propranolol
    c. If necessary, DC cardioversion

### Heart Block

1. 1° AV block, Type I
   2° block (Wenckebach)
    a. Atropine
    b. Isoproterenol
2. Type II 2° block, complete heart block
    a. Temporary pacemaker
    b. Permanent pacemaker

### Ventricular Arrhythmias

1. Ventricular premature contractions
    a. Lidocaine
    b. Procainamide or disopyramide
    c. Bretyllium
    d. Quinidine
2. Ventricular tachycardia
    a. DC cardioversion
    b. Lidocaine
    c. Procainamide
    d. Bretyllium
    e. Quinidine

*Verapamil is becoming the drug of choice for reentrant arrhythmias involving the AV node and for immediately controlling the ventricular rate in atrial fibrillation and flutter.

3. Ventricular fibrillation
   a. DC cardioversion and cardiopulmonary resuscitation
   b. Lidocaine or procainamide
   c. Bretyllium
4. Digitalis-induced arrhythmias
   a. For atrial tachycardia with block
      i. Phenytoin (plus KCL)
      ii. Propranolol
   b. For VPCs
      i. Lidocaine (plus KCL)
      ii. Phenytoin or propranolol

## ANTIARRHYTHMIC AGENTS

### Group I: Quinidine, procainamide, disopyramide

Electrical effects
    i. Suppress automaticity
    ii. Increase refractory period
    iii. Increase duration of action potential
    iv. Decrease conduction velocity
    v. Vagolytic
1. Quinidine
    a. ECG effects
        i. Prolongs QT interval
        ii. Prolongs QRS complex
        iii. Reduces T wave voltage
        iv. U waves
    b. Side effects
        i. GI distress (especially diarrhea)
        ii. Paroxysmal ventricular tachycardia (heralded by lengthening QT)
        iii. Hypotension
        iv. Exacerbates congestive heart failure
        v. Drug fever, rash
        vi. Thrombocytopenia
        vii. Granulomatous hepatitis
        viii. Arthralgias
        ix. Pleuritis and pericarditis
        x. Cinchonism (vertigo, tinnitus, headache, fever, visual disturbances)
        xi. Increases digoxin level when used concomitantly
    Half-life: 5–7 hours; elimination: hepatic and renal
2. Procainamide
    a. ECG effects
        i. Prolongs QT interval (less than quinidine)
        ii. Prolongs QRS complex
        iii. Reduces T wave voltage
    b. Side effects
        i. Exacerbates congestive heart failure
        ii. Lupuslike syndrome
        iii. GI distress
        iv. Drug fever, rash
    Half-life: 3 hours; elimination: hepatic and renal

3. Disopyramide
   a. ECG effect: prolongs QT interval
   b. Side effects
      i. Paroxysmal ventricular tachycardia
      ii. Dry mouth
      iii. Urinary retention
      iv. Constipation
      v. Blurred vision
      vi. Abdominal pain
      vii. Hypotension
      viii. Exacerbation of congestive heart failure (the most severe negative inotrope)

   Half-life: 5–6 hours; elimination: hepatic and renal

## Group II: Lidocaine, phenytoin

Electrical effects
      i. Suppress automaticity
      ii. Decrease refractory period
      iii. Decrease duration of action potential
      iv. Increase conduction velocity

1. Lidocaine
   a. ECG effects: None
   b. Side effects: neurologic—agitation, confusion, seizures, coma

   Half-life: 1.5 hours (IV, after initial loading); elimination: hepatic

2. Phenytoin
   a. ECG effect: shortens QT interval
   b. Side effects: See list "Side Effects of Some Common Anti-convulsants"

   Half-life: 4–6 hours; elimination: hepatic

## Group III: Propranolol

Electrical effects
      i. Suppresses automaticity
      ii. Increases refractory period
      iii. No effect on duration of action potential
      iv. Decreases conduction velocity
      v. β-Blockade
   a. ECG effects
      i. Prolongs PR interval
      ii. Shortens QT interval

## ANTIARRHYTHMIC AGENTS *(cont.)*

  b. Side effects
      i. Sinus bradycardia
      ii. Exacerbates congestive heart failure
      iii. Exacerbates diabetes mellitus
      iv. Bronchial asthma
      v. Drug fever, rash
      vi. GI distress
      vii. Blood dyscrasias
      viii. Precipitates angina, arrhythmias
      ix. CNS effects (depression, drowsiness, disorientation, visual disturbances)
  Half-life: 3–6 hours; elimination: hepatic

### Group IV: Bretyllium

  Electrical effects
      i. Suppresses automaticity
      ii. Increases refractory period
      iii. Increases duration of action potential
      iv. No effect on conduction velocity
      v. Adrenergic stimulation
  a. ECG effect: prolongs QT interval
  b. Side effects
      i. Orthostatic hypotension
      ii. GI distress
      iii. Skin rash
      iv. Emotional lability
      v. Exacerbates dig-toxic arrhythmias
  Half-life: 4–18 hours; elimination: renal

### Group V: Verapamil

  Electrical effects
      i. Inhibits calcium flux across cardiac cells
      ii. Slows conduction through AV node
  a. ECG effects: None
  b. Side effects
      i. Hypotension and bradycardia
      ii. Exacerbates congestive heart failure
      iii. GI distress
      iv. Headache
      v. Dizziness
  Half-life: 1 hour (when given IV); elimination: hepatic

## CONGESTIVE HEART FAILURE: ESTABLISHING THE DIAGNOSIS

### History

Questions should be directed at determining (1) the underlying etiology of the heart failure, (2) the immediate precipitant(s) of worsening failure, (3) current respiratory and exertional symptoms as an indication of the severity of failure, and (4) predominance of left- versus right-sided symptoms.

1. Underlying etiologies of heart failure
   a. Ischemic heart disease
   b. Valvular disease
   c. Cardiomyopathy
   d. Myocarditis
   e. Hypertension
   f. Pericardial disease
   g. Rarely, high-output states without any underlying cardiac abnormality (hyperthyroidism, anemia, AV fistulae, Paget's disease)
2. Precipitants of worsening left ventricle failure
   a. Worsened contractility
      i. Further structural damage to myocardium (e.g., new infarction)
      ii. Decreased $O_2$ supply (hypoxia, anemia, pulmonary embolism)
      iii. Increased $O_2$ demand (fever, infection, thyrotoxicosis, stress)
      iv. Negative inotropic forces (acidosis, too little digoxin, antiarrhythmic drugs)
   b. Increased afterload (volume or pressure overload)
      i. Noncompliance with diet or diuretic prescription
      ii. I.V. fluid or salt overload
      iii. Decreased fluid or salt excretion (e.g., renal failure, mineralocorticoid use)
      iv. Worsened valvular dysfunction (aortic or mitral regurgitation)
      v. Hypertension
   c. Decreased preload (causing low output failure)
      i. Worsened mitral stenosis
      ii. Ineffective filling (atrial fibrillation, tachyarrhythmias)
      iii. Worsened restrictive cardiomyopathy or pericardial effusions
   d. Rate dependent decrease in cardiac output (bradycardia)
3. Symptoms
   a. The cardinal symptom of left-sided heart failure is *dyspnea,*

## CONGESTIVE HEART FAILURE:
## ESTABLISHING THE DIAGNOSIS *(cont.)*

progressing from dyspnea on exertion to orthopnea and paroxysmal nocturnal dyspnea. Peripheral edema can result from a low output state, stimulating the kidneys to retain sodium and water.

b. The cardinal symptoms of right-sided heart failure are jugular venous distension, a positive hepatojugular reflex, hepatomegaly, ascites, and peripheral edema.

c. Other symptoms include fatigue, weakness, nocturia, impaired consciousness, abdominal fullness and various gastrointestinal complaints.

### *Differential Diagnosis of Dyspnea*

1. Congestive heart failure
2. Chronic obstructive pulmonary disease
3. Pulmonary emboli
4. Pulmonary hypertension
5. Aspiration
6. Pulmonary parenchymal diseases (infection, neoplasia, etc)
7. Disease of chest wall or respiratory musculature
8. Hyperventilation syndrome
9. Anemia
10. Thyrotoxicosis

## Physical Examination: Common Findings

1. General appearance: patient may be acutely anxious and in obvious distress, or may only note discomfort when asked to exert himself or lie down.
2. Vital signs: tachycardia, tachypnea, and slight hypertension are common.
3. Vascular: elevated neck veins; pulsus alternans (best tested by palpation of the femoral artery).
4. Cardiac: $S_3$ gallop ($S_4$ may also be present); paradoxical splitting of $S_2$ ($P_2$ may be louder than $A_2$); murmurs may be present, either reflecting underlying pathology or secondary to ventricular dilation (regurgitant murmurs).
5. Pulmonary: moist rales over lung bases (often with dullness to percussion); pink, frothy sputum (if onset of pulmonary edema is acute).
6. Abdominal: hepatomegaly; liver is tender; ascites; positive hepatojugular reflex (with mild right heart failure).
7. Extremities: skin is cold and pale; digits cyanotic; peripheral edema (appears first in dependent areas, usually the feet and ankles in ambulatory patients).

8. CNS: sluggish sensorium, confusion in extreme low output states.

## Laboratory

The following studies should be ordered:

1. CBC
2. Serum electrolytes
3. BUN, creatinine
4. Liver function tests
5. Urinalysis
6. ECG (to look for new infarction, arrhythmias)
7. CXR

## Radiographic Findings

1. Pulmonary venous distention—most easily seen in upper hilus on right side; correlates with PCW pressure at 15–18 mm Hg.
2. Interstitial pulmonary edema—Kerley A lines represent edematous interlobular septa in upper lung fields; Kerley B lines represent septal edema in periphery of lower lung fields. Perivascular cutting denotes perivascular edema; correlates with PCW pressure at 19–25 mm Hg.
3. Alveolar pulmonary edema correlates with PCW pressure > 25 mm Hg.

   Further work-up should be guided by the results of these studies, the history, and physical examination.

## Management

1. If an underlying etiology has been identified, treat with specific measures.
2. Treat any remediable precipitant(s) with specific measures.
3. General therapy for heart failure
   a. Salt restriction (<2,000 mg/day)
   b. Weight loss if the patient is overweight
   c. Bed rest with the head elevated
   d. Improve contractility with a cardiac glycoside
   e. Decrease preload using venodilators—nitrates (isosorbide dinitrate [Isordil] and nitroglycerin ointment). Afterload can be reduced with hydralazine. Unloading agents are generally reserved for patients not responding to digoxin and diuretics.
   f. Treat pulmonary edema with morphine, oxygen, diuretics, rotating tourniquets, and, rarely, phlebotomy.

## CARDIAC GLYCOSIDES

1. Mechanism of action: Improve cardiac contractility, presumably by increasing myocardial intracellular calcium stores through inhibitory effect on the membrane-bound sodium–potassium ATPase
2. Pharmacokinetics of digoxin
   a. Peak plasma level (after an oral dose): 2–3 hours
   b. Maximal effect: 4–6 hours
   c. Percent bound to protein: 25%
   d. Half-life: 1–2 days
   e. Elimination: renal
3. Use in congestive heart failure
   a. Usually beneficial in heart failure resulting from valvular disease, ischemic disease, congenital heart disease, hypertension, and supraventricular arrhythmias
   b. May be beneficial in heart failure resulting from cardiomyopathy and myocarditis
   c. Not helpful in heart failure resulting from pericardial disease and high output states
4. Toxicity
   a. The dose must be individually titrated for each patient (a typical daily oral maintenance dose of digoxin ranges from 0.125 mg to 0.50 mg (occasionally more in atrial fibrillation with a rapid ventricular response)
   b. Before giving the drug
      i. Obtain a baseline ECG
      ii. Correct any electrolyte imbalances (hypokalemia, in particular, predisposes to digitalis toxicity)
      iii. Assess the patient's renal function
   c. Toxic side effects
      i. Gastrointestinal: nausea, vomiting, anorexia, abdominal distress
      ii. CNS: altered vision (blurring, photophobia, disturbed color vision), drowsiness, depression
      iii. Cardiac: heart block, arrhythmias (especially ventricular ectopy, junctional arrhythmias, sinus bradycardia, PAT with block)
   d. Monitor the patient with
      i. Serial ECGs
      ii. Serum digoxin levels
      iii. Subjective response and physical examination

e. If toxic effects supervene
  i. Discontinue the drug
  ii. Obtain an ECG and a serum level
  iii. Correct hypokalemia and any other metabolic disturbances
  iv. Treat toxic arrhythmias with phenytoin or lidocaine: treat bradycardia with atropine
f. Electrical cardioversion is extremely hazardous in a patient with digitalis toxicity, since it may precipitate lethal arrhythmias.

# FACTORS AFFECTING DIGITALIS BLOOD LEVELS*

1. Factors causing low drug levels
   a. Decreased absorption
      i. Decreased gut circulation secondary to congestive heart failure
      ii. Concomitant administration of antacids or kaolin–pectin compounds
      iii. Cellulose-containing laxatives that bind digoxin
   b. Increased metabolism: phenobarbital and phenylbutazone, which cause increased digitoxin metabolism
2. Factors causing high drug levels
   a. Decreased metabolism
      i. Renal insufficiency, causing decreased digoxin excretion
      ii. Hepatic insufficiency, causing decreased digitoxin metabolism
   b. Drug interactions: concurrent administration of quinidine
3. Factors enhancing potential for myocardial toxicity
   a. Electrolyte abnormalities: decreased $K^+$, $Mg^{++}$; increased $Ca^{++}$
   b. Hypoxemia
   c. Acidosis

*Blood levels interact with myocardial uptake of the drug to determine whether the drug effects are suboptimal, therapeutic, or toxic. Absolute levels without consideration of myocardial interaction are less helpful.

## VALVULAR DISEASE

### Mitral Stenosis

1. Etiology: Rheumatic fever (50–60% of patients give a positive history of acute rheumatic fever). Congenital lesions are far less common.
2. Natural history: The earliest symptom, dyspnea on exertion, appears 15 to 20 years after the episode of acute rheumatic fever. Symptoms usually appear when the valve orifice has narrowed to less than 1.5 cm² (normal 3–4). In most patients, progressive pulmonary edema leads to worsening dyspnea (orthopnea and paroxysmal nocturnal dyspnea), cough, and fatigue. In some patients, however, pulmonary vasoconstriction spares the patient from pulmonary edema, but at the expense of cor pulmonale and right heart failure. Without treatment, incapacity frequently develops within 5 to 10 years after the onset of symptoms. Manifestations at the time of diagnosis may include hemoptysis (early in the course), atrial fibrillation, and systemic embolization. Ten percent of patients experience chest pain.
3. Physiology: left atrial pressures rise to maintain cardiac output. This causes pulmonary venous pressures to rise, leading to pulmonary edema (unless there is concurrent pulmonary vasoconstriction). Eventually, the cardiac output itself can no longer be maintained.
4. Cardiac exam.
   a. There is a rumbling diastolic murmur, best heard at the apex, often without significant radiation.
   b. The murmur is most prominent after exercise and with the patient in the left lateral decubitus position.
   c. The murmur is unaffected by or slightly decreased with inspiration (the murmur of tricuspid stenosis increases) and increased with amyl nitrite (the Austin-Flint murmur decreases).
   d. In patients with normal sinus rhythm, there is a presystolic accentuation.
   e. There is a loud, snapping $S_1$.
   f. An opening snap is heard early in diastole unless the valve is fixed.
   g. $S_3$ and $S_4$ gallops are rarely heard.
5. Other findings:
   a. The "mitral facies"—malar flush, cyanosis of the lips—is uncommon.
   b. Rales may be heard.

## VALVULAR DISEASE *(cont.)*

   c. Patients may develop the full-blown picture of right heart failure (peripheral edema, ascites, etc) with the murmurs of pulmonic regurgitation (Graham Steell) and tricuspid regurgitation.

6. ECG
   a. Large notched P waves of left atrial enlargement may appear.
   b. Atrial fibrillation frequently occurs.
7. Chest x-ray
   a. Enlarged left atrium may be evidenced by convexity of the left upper cardiac margin, a double convexity on the right, and posterior displacement of a barium-filled esophagus.
   b. Upper lobe pulmonary vessels are more pronounced than lower lobe (reversal of the usual pattern).
   c. Kerley B lines appear at the lung bases (representing interstitial edema).
   d. Eventual right ventricular enlargement and dilation of central pulmonary arteries are evident.

## Mitral Regurgitation

1. Etiology: Rheumatic fever, mitral valve prolapse, papillary muscle dysfunction (e.g., as a result of dilation due to congestive heart failure) or rupture (e.g., as a result of infarction), ruptured chordae tendineae, endocarditis, cardiomyopathy, idiopathic mitral valve calcification.
2. Natural history: The lesion is generally well tolerated, and symptoms of failure—fatigue and dyspnea—develop slowly and late in the disease course. The incidence of pulmonary edema, hemoptysis, and embolization is low compared to that of mitral stenosis. Atrial fibrillation can develop, but is also less common than in mitral stenosis.

      Acute mitral regurgitation can result from rupture of the papillary muscles or chordae tendinae, and may occasionally occur in patients with mitral valve prolapse. Shock and acute pulmonary edema ensue.
3. Physiology: Ejection of the excess volume into the low-resistance left atrium spares the left ventricle the excessive overwork encountered with equal volumes in aortic regurgitation. Nevertheless, the left atrium and, eventually, the left ventricle enlarge.
4. Cardiac exam:
   a. A blowing, holosystolic murmur best heard at the apex and generally radiating to the axilla (the murmur of a ventral septal defect (VSD) is harsh).

b. The murmur is unaffected by or slightly decreased with inspiration (the murmur of tricuspid regurgitation increases and is best heard at the lower left sternal border) and decreased with amyl nitrite (the murmur of aortic stenosis increases).
   c. $S_1$ is soft or absent.
   d. $P_2$ is loud if there is pulmonary hypertension.
   e. A loud $S_3$ is common, and may be followed by a short diastolic rumble.
   f. The prolapsed valve produces midsystolic clicks, and the murmur tends to be more late systolic.
   g. A strong apical beat may be felt.
5. Other findings:
   a. The carotid pulse is abrupt and collapsing (with a VSD it is sometimes bisferiens; with aortic stenosis it is typically tardus et parvus).
   b. Pulmonary rales may be heard.
   c. Evidence of right heart failure may be present, but left heart failure usually predominates.
6. ECG:
   a. Broad, notched P waves of atrial enlargement.
   b. Left axis deviation.
7. Chest x-ray:
   a. Enlarged left atrium and left ventricle.
   b. Mitral valve calcification.
8. Mitral valve prolapse:
   a. Redundant mitral valve tissue is present in 5–10% of young healthy females.
   b. It is generally benign, but sudden death may occur. The most common associated symptoms are chest pain, fatigue, dyspnea, and palpitations.
   c. Midsystolic clicks are best heard at the apex; standing prolongs the murmur and moves the clicks closer to $S_1$; squatting shortens the murmur and moves the clicks closer to $S_2$.

## Aortic Stenosis

1. Etiology: Rheumatic fever (virtually always with concurrent mitral valve involvement), congenitally bicuspid valve (isolated aortic stenosis).
2. Natural history: Symptoms don't appear until the degree of stenosis becomes very severe (valve area less than 1.0 cm²; normal, 2.6–3.5). Eventually, the increased oxygen demands of the hypertrophied myocardium lead to angina, syncope (usually exertional), and symptoms of left heart failure. Without surgery, life expectancy following the onset of angina is five years, syn-

## VALVULAR DISEASE *(cont.)*

cope three years, and heart failure two years. Many patients die a sudden death.

3. Physiology: The left ventricle hypertrophies to maintain cardiac output against a narrowing orifice. An increasing pressure gradient develops across the valve, producing a murmur. The quality of the murmur (see below) does not correlate with the severity of stenosis. Better measures are the carotid upstroke and the delay of $A_2$.

4. Cardiac exam:
   a. A rough, low-pitched, crescendo-decrescendo murmur best heard at the base and radiating to the carotids (the murmur of ASH is less harsh and maximal at the left lower sternal border or apex).
   b. The murmur is decreased with inspiration (the murmur of pulmonary stenosis is increased) and increased with amyl nitrate (the murmur of mitral regurgitation is decreased).
   c. $A_2$ is decreased or absent.
   d. $S_2$ may be paradoxically split.
   e. $S_3$ and $S_4$ gallops may be present.
   f. A systolic ejection sound may be heard; it diminishes with progressive calcification and is unchanged by inspiration (the ejection sound of pulmonary stenosis decreases with inspiration).
   g. The benign ejection murmur of old age is less rough, less intense, and transmits to the apex.

5. Other findings: Carotid pulse is tardus et parvus, and a systolic thrill may be palpated (the carotid pulse in patients with the benign ejection murmur of old age is usually normal).

6. ECG: Left ventricular strain—increased QRS voltage, ST depression and T wave inversion in I, AVL, and left precordial leads.

7. Chest x-ray:
   a. A calcified valve is seen.
   b. Aortic root may be enlarged (poststenotic dilatation).
   c. Concentric left ventricular hypertrophy may only be apparent as a rounding at the apex.

### Aortic Regurgitation

1. Etiology: Rheumatic fever, connective tissue disorders, endocarditis, syphilis, dissecting aneurysm, distortions of the aortic root (as, e.g., in Marfan's syndrome and ankylosing spondylitis).

2. Natural history: Many patients experience no symptoms for several decades. As the volume load on the left ventricle in-

creases, however, angina and symptoms of left heart failure eventually appear. Progression is rapid without surgical intervention.

Acute aortic regurgitation can result from trauma or endocarditis. The normal-sized left ventricle cannot handle the suddenly increased volume load, and severe pulmonary edema and failure develop rapidly.

3. Physiology: Volume overload of the left ventricle causes hypertrophy, dilatation, and eventual failure. The fall in cardiac output and increased myocardial oxygen demands are responsible for the symptoms.
4. Cardiac exam:
   a. A high-pitched (occasionally harsh or musical), blowing, decrescendo diastolic murmur best heard at the left sternal border (at the right sternal border with disease of the aortic root).
   b. The murmur is best heard in full expiration with the patient leaning forward.
   c. The murmur decreases with amyl nitrite (the murmur of mitral stenosis increases, while that of pulmonic regurgation increases or is unaffected).
   d. $S_1$ and $S_2$ are usually normal.
   e. An $S_3$ gallop may be present.
   f. A second, rumbling murmur—the Austin-Flint murmur—may also be heard; it is due to the regurgitant stream striking the mitral valve and resembles mitral stenosis. The Austin-Flint murmur also diminishes with amyl nitrite, unlike that of mitral stenosis.
5. Other findings:
   a. Bounding, waterhammer, or bisferiens carotid pulse.
   b. Capillary pulsations in nail beds.
   c. "Pistol shot" bruits over femoral arteries.
   d. Widened pulse pressure.
   e. Pulsation of uvula, head, liver, and spleen with each heartbeat.
6. ECG: Left ventricular strain.
7. Chest x-ray:
   a. Left ventricle may be considerably enlarged.
   b. There is dilation of the aortic root.

## Right-sided Valvular Lesions

Tricuspid and pulmonic valvular lesions are difficult to diagnose and are frequently overlooked. Symptomatically, they are generally well tolerated for many years. When symptoms do appear, they are those of right-sided failure and diminished cardiac output. On examination, the presence of right-sided failure may be signalled by an $S_3$

## VALVULAR DISEASE *(cont.)*

gallop that increases in intensity with inspiration. ECG and chest x-ray findings mirror those of their left-sided counterparts.

1. Tricuspid stenosis
   a. Etiology: rheumatic fever (almost always with coexistent mitral stenosis); less common causes include congenital lesions, carcinoid syndrome, and atrial tumors.
   b. Cardiac exam:
      i. A rumbling, diastolic murmur is heard at the lower left sternal border; the murmur increases with inspiration and amyl nitrite; if atrial fibrillation has not developed, the murmur has a presystolic accentuation.
      ii. There is an opening snap.
      iii. There are large jugular "A" waves.
      iv. No right ventricular heave can be felt.
2. Tricuspid regurgitation
   a. Etiology: Dilation of the right ventricle is due to right-sided failure (most often secondary to mitral valvular disease or pulmonary hypertension); other less common causes include rheumatic fever, papillary muscle or chordae tendinae rupture, endocarditis (leading cause of isolated tricuspid regurgitation), cardiomyopathy, and carcinoid syndrome.
   b. Cardiac exam:
      i. A high-pitched, holosystolic murmur is heard at the lower left sternal border; the murmur increases with inspiration and amyl nitrite.
      ii. There are large jugular "V" waves.
      iii. Atrial fibrillation is very common.
3. Pulmonic Stenosis
   a. Etiology: congenital lesions and rheumatic fever; rarely, carcinoid syndrome.
   b. Cardiac exam:
      i. A harsh, crescendo-decrescendo systolic murmur is heard at the upper left sternal border; the murmur increases with inspiration and amyl nitrite.
      ii. The murmur of a VSD is very similar; however, in a VSD, $S_2$ is generally normally split, while in pulmonic stenosis $S_2$ is widely split and $P_2$ may be soft.
      iii. There is an ejection sound.
      iv. There are large jugular "A" waves.
      v. A right ventricular heave can be felt.

4. Pulmonic Regurgitation
   a. Etiology: dilation of the valvular ring due to pulmonary hypertension; less common causes include endocarditis, rheumatic fever, trauma, syphilis, and carcinoid syndrome.
   b. Cardiac exam:
      i. A high-pitched, blowing diastolic murmur is heard at the upper left sternal border; the murmur increases with inspiration and may increase or remain unchanged with amyl nitrite.
      ii. There is an ejection sound.
      iii. $S_2$ is widely split.
      iv. A right ventricular heave can be felt (unlike tricuspid regurgitation).

## FACTORS ALTERING THE MURMUR OF ASYMMETRIC SEPTAL HYPERTROPHY

### Factors Enhancing the Murmur

1. Diminished ventricular size
   a. Valsalva maneuver
   b. Standing
   c. Tachycardia
   d. Amyl nitrate
   e. Vasodilator drugs
2. Increased contractility
   a. Premature beats ("postextrasystolic potentiation")
   b. Digitalis
   c. $\beta$-Adrenergic drugs (e.g., isoproterenol)

### Factors decreasing the murmur

1. Increased ventricular size
   a. Leg raising
   b. Sitting or squatting
   c. Bradycardia
   d. $\alpha$-Adrenergic drugs (e.g., phenylephrine)
2. Decreased contractility: $\beta$-adrenergic blockade (e.g., propranolol)

## CARDIOMYOPATHY

### Classification: Congestive

*Common Causes:* idiopathic, alcoholic, peripartal, infectious (usually Coxsackie B virus), toxic (neoplastic drugs)

*Pathology:* enlarged heart with fibrosis and mild hypertrophy

*Major hemodynamic features:* diminished contractility, leading to poor cardiac output and elevated venous pressure

*Clinical Manifestations:* congestive heart failure, usually predominantly left-sided (causing dyspnea, fatigue and peripheral edema), arrhythmias, pulmonary and systemic emboli

*Physical Exam:* $S_3$, $S_4$ gallops; mild to severe cardiomegaly, regurgitant murmurs

*Prognosis:* Five-year average survival after onset of symptoms, although some patients survive much longer

### Classification: Restrictive

*Common Causes:* amyloidosis, hemochromatosis (other infiltrative diseases are much less common), endomyocardial fibrosis (in equatorial regions)

*Pathology:* amyloid deposits in and around myocardial cells

*Major hemodynamic features:* "stiff," noncompliant heart, leading to elevated diastolic pressures

*Clinical Manifestations:* congestive heart failure, usually predominantly right-sided (causing ascites, hepatomegaly), arrhythmias, especially dig-toxic arrhythmias; picture mimics constrictive pericarditis

*Physical Exam:* mild cardiomegaly, Kussmaul's sign (inspiratory increase in venous pressure), $S_3$, $S_4$ gallops

*Prognosis:* three- to six-year average survival

## CARDIOMYOPATHY *(cont.)*

### Classification: Hypertrophic

*Common Causes:* asymmetric septal hypertrophy (idiopathic)

*Pathology:* hypertrophied septum filled with enlarged, disorganized muscle bundles

*Major hemodynamic features:* stiffened, noncompliant ventricles; outflow may be unimpeded or obstructed (fixed or labile obstruction)

*Clinical manifestations:* syncope (usually with exercise), angina, sudden death, arrhythmias, congestive heart failure

*Physical Exam:* mild cardiomegaly, $S_3$, $S_4$ gallops, murmur of outflow obstruction, murmur of mitral regurgitation

*Prognosis:* Most patients do well for many years, although there is an increased risk of sudden death

## COMMON CAUSES OF PERICARDITIS

1. Infectious
   a. Viral (usually Coxsackie B)
   b. Bacterial (almost any organism, more often by local spread than septicemia)
   c. Tuberculosis
   d. Fungal (generally in immunosuppressed patients)
   e. Parasitic
2. Immunologic
   a. Autoimmune disorders (SLE, scleroderma, rheumatoid arthritis)
   b. Vasculitides (polyarteritis nodosa)
   c. Drug reactions (SLE-like syndromes associated with procainamide, hydralazine, isoniazid, and others)
   d. Acute rheumatic fever
   e. Serum sickness
   f. Postmyocardial infarction (Dressler's) syndrome
   g. (?) Postcardiotomy syndrome
3. Metabolic
   a. Uremia
   b. Myxedema
4. Myocardial infarction
5. Dissecting aneurysm
6. Trauma
7. Irradiation
8. Neoplastic disease
   a. Primary mesothelioma (rare)
   b. Metastatic spread (usually lung, breast, lymphoma, or melanoma)

## DIAGNOSIS OF PERICARDIAL DISEASE

1. Acute pericarditis
   a. Symptoms: chest pain, sometimes referred to the neck or shoulders, typically stabbing, affected by both respiration and position
   b. Signs: friction rub, best heard along the left sternal border during forced expiration while the patient is leaning forward; in its full expression the rub has three components corresponding with atrial contraction, ventricular contraction, and ventricular filling
   c. ECG: ST elevation, concave upward; T wave abnormalities (flattening, inversion); supraventricular arrhythmias
   d. Chest x-ray: Heart is typically enlarged and globular (if there is a pericardial effusion); frequently, there are concomitant pulmonary infiltrates or a pleural effusion
2. Development of pericardial tamponade
   a. Symptoms: cyanosis, dyspnea, agitation, or loss of consciousness
   b. Signs: tachycardia, pulsus paradoxus, diminished blood pressure, jugular venous distention, distant heart sounds
3. Chronic constrictive pericarditis (may develop from acute pericarditis or without any evidence of an acute episode)
   a. Symptoms: ascites, edema, hepatomegaly
   b. Signs: elevated venous pressures with a pronounced "Y" descent in the jugular pulse, Kussmaul's sign, an early diastolic knock, low serum albumin (protein-losing enteropathy)
   c. ECG: low voltage, nonspecific ST and T wave changes, irregular P waves, atrial fibrillation
   d. Chest x-ray: Heart may appear small, 50% reveal pericardial calcification

## COR PULMONALE: CAUSES

Cor pulmonale is defined as enlargement of the right ventricle due to pulmonary hypertension.

### Important Causes of Pulmonary Hypertension

1. Loss of pulmonary vasculature
   a. Multiple pulmonary emboli
   b. Pulmonary thrombosis (e.g., due to sickle cell crisis)
   c. Primary pulmonary hypertension
   d. Inflammatory and fibrosing diseases (including SLE, scleroderma, polyarteritis nodosa, sarcoidosis, and the pneumoconioses)
2. Pulmonary vasoconstriction resulting from hypoxia and acidosis
   a. Chronic obstructive pulmonary disease
   b. Impaired ventilatory drive (Ondine's curse)
   c. Sleep-apnea syndrome
   d. Pickwickian syndrome
   e. Kyphoscoliosis
   f. Myasthenia gravis and other neuromuscular disorders
3. Increased pulmonary venous pressure
   a. Mitral stenosis
   b. Pulmonary venous disease
4. Increased pulmonary flow (pressure elevation is generally mild): large left-to-right shunts (e.g., patent ductus arteriosus and ventricular septal defect)

## COR PULMONALE: DIAGNOSIS AND ASSESSMENT

1. Symptoms: early—nonspecific, usually no more than modest fatigue or weakness; occasional hemoptysis; late—RUQ fullness, edema, dyspnea
2. Physical exam
   a. Early signs, associated with right ventricular hypertrophy
      i. Loud $P_2$, often palpable
      ii. Right ventricular heave
      iii. Large jugular "a" waves
      iv. Short pulmonic ejection murmur
      v. Soft pulmonic regurgitant murmur
   b. Late signs, associated with right ventricular dilation and failure
      i. Large jugular "v" waves
      ii. Systemic venous congestion—peripheral edema, ascites, hepatomegaly, elevated neck veins
      iii. Murmur of tricuspid regurgitation
      iv. Right-sided $S_3$ (increases with inspiration)
3. Chest x-ray
   a. Right atrial and right ventricular enlargement
   b. Enlarged hilar vessels with avascular periphery
4. ECG
   a. Changes most specific to cor pulmonale include large R waves and inverted T waves in leads $V_1$ and $V_2$
   b. Suggestive changes include peaked P waves in leads II, III, and AVF, right axis deviation, and right bundle branch block.

## CLINICAL MANIFESTATIONS OF INFECTIOUS ENDOCARDITIS

1. General: fever,* weakness,* malaise,* chills, sweats, anorexia, weight loss
2. Cardiopulmonary
   a. Heart murmur,* changing murmur, new murmur, chest pain, myocardial infarction, congestive heart failure
   b. Dyspnea,* cough, pulmonary emboli, pneumonia, hemoptysis
3. Genitourinary: hematuria,* proteinuria,* flank pain, renal failure
4. Gastrointestinal: abdominal pain, mesenteric vascular occlusion, abnormal liver function tests, nausea, vomiting
5. Hematologic: splenomegaly,* anemia, leukocytosis, thrombocytopenia, disseminated intravascular coagulation (DIC)
6. Neurologic: cerebral infarction,* mycotic aneurysms, microscopic brain abscesses, meningitis, subarachnoid hemorrhage, seizures
7. Musculoskeletal: arthralgias, myalgias, back pain, clubbing, osteomyelitis
8. Dermatologic: petechiae,* splinter hemorrhages, Osler's nodes, Janeway lesions
9. Ocular: Roth's spots

Note: The most common presenting symptoms are indicated with *.

## MAJOR CAUSES OF HYPERTENSION

1. Essential hypertension: at least 90% of all cases of hypertension
2. Secondary hypertension
   a. Renal
      i. Renal artery stenosis
      ii. Renal parenchymal disease
      iii. Renin-producing tumors
   b. Adrenal
      i. Primary hyperaldosteronism (Conn's syndrome, idiopathic)
      ii. Cushing's syndrome
      iii. Pheochromocytoma
   c. Cardiovascular: coarctation of the aorta
   d. Use of oral contraceptives, steroids, or amphetamines

## HYPERTENSION: INITIAL EVALUATION

Hypertension is diagnosed when two separate measurements of a patient's blood pressure exceed values associated with a 50% increase in mortality. For men younger than 45, this value is 130/90; for men older than 45 this value is 140/95; for women of all ages this value is 160/95. All patients with newly diagnosed hypertension should receive the following limited initial workup (as a minimum):

1. History
   a. Family history of hypertension?
   b. Age of onset?
   c. Use of salt? Dietary habits?
   d. Exercise?
   e. History of heart disease, lipid disorder, diabetes, gout, or renal disorder?
   f. Symptoms of pheochromocytoma or hyperthyroidism?
   g. Use of agents associated with hypertension (steroids, hormones, adrenergic stimulants)?
2. Physical exam
   a. Look for clues to etiology (obesity? asymmetric pulses? stigmata of chronic renal insufficiency? hyperthyroidism or Cushing's syndrome?)
   b. Evaluate evidence of end organ damage (hypertensive retinopathy? cardiomyopathy or congestive failure? signs of renal insufficiency?)
3. Laboratory evaluation
   a. Serum electrolytes.
   b. Serum creatinine and BUN.
   c. Urinalysis.
   d. ECG.
   e. Chest x-ray.

A fasting blood sugar and serum lipids may also prove helpful.

If there are no findings in the history, physical exam, or above laboratory studies to suggest a possible secondary cause of hypertension (e.g., onset of severe hypertension in young patient without family history, sudden onset of severe hypertension in older patient, hypertension associated with symptoms suggestive of renal or adrenal disease), one can initiate therapy assuming the diagnosis of essential hypertension. If therapy is unsuccessful, or if there are positive features in the initial workup, a more comprehensive workup is required to seek a cause of secondary hypertension.

## SECONDARY HYPERTENSION: DIFFERENTIAL DIAGNOSTIC CLUES AND WORKUP

1. Renal artery stenosis
   a. Signs and symptoms: bruit over flank or epigastrium
   b. Laboratory
      i. Best screen: rapid sequence IV pyelogram (most sensitive criterion is delayed appearance of dye in affected kidney; other criteria include delay in dye emptying and shortening of affected kidney >1.5 cm). Also useful—renal scan, looking for delayed perfusion, and plasma renin activity (PRA)
      ii. Confirmation: renal arteriography and selective renal vein renin assays (a ratio of >1.5 is considered diagnostic)
2. Renal parenchymal disease (usually chronic pyelonephritis, glomerulonephritis)
   a. Signs and symptoms: fatigue, anorexia, pallor, nausea, edema; polycystic kidneys may be palpable
   b. Laboratory
      i. Best screen: elevated serum creatinine and BUN, and abnormal urinary sediment
      ii. Confirmation: creatinine clearance, renal scan, renal biopsy
3. Renin-producing tumor
   a. Laboratory: arteriography and selective renin assays
4. Primary hyperaldosteronism
   a. Signs and symptoms: polyuria, polydipsia, weakness, paresthesias; hypertension is usually mild
   b. Laboratory
      i. Best screen: hypokalemia, mild hypernatremia
      ii. Confirmation: elevated serum aldosterone, decreased plasma renin activity
5. Cushing's syndrome
   a. Signs and symptoms: moon facies, truncal obesity, hirsutism, pigmented striae, easy bruising, weakness, backache, sexual dysfunction
   b. Laboratory
      i. Best screen: dexamethasone (1 mg) suppression test
      ii. Confirmation: increased urinary-free cortisol or 17-hydroxycorticosteroids

6. Pheochromocytoma
   a. Signs and symptoms: palpitations, flushing, headache, sweating, weight loss, dizziness, nervousness, abdominal pain, tachycardia, orthostatic hypotension
   b. Laboratory
      i. Best screen: 24-hour urine collection for catecholamine metabolites (metanephrine or VMA)
      ii. Confirmation: localize tumor with ultrasound or CT scan
7. Coarctation of the aorta
   a. Signs and symptoms: often no symptoms, others experience headache and exertional claudication; key finding is diminished pulses (and, frequently, underdeveloped muscle mass) in lower extremities; systolic murmur may be heard in back between scapulae; intercostal pulsations may be felt
   b. Laboratory
      i. Chest x-ray may show rib notching, classic "3" sign
      ii. Confirmation: aortic angiography
8. Use of oral contraceptives
   a. Signs and symptoms: hypertension is mild
   b. Laboratory: elevated renin substrate

## OPHTHALMOSCOPIC GRADING OF HYPERTENSIVE–ARTERIOSCLEROTIC RETINOPATHY

1. Grade I
   a. Slight arteriolar narrowing (A:V = 1:2)
   b. Slight AV nicking
2. Grade II
   a. More pronounced arteriolar narrowing
   b. Moderate AV nicking (A:V = 1:3)
   c. Geographic irregularities: AV crossings at right angles
3. Grade III
   a. Copper wire arterioles
   b. Marked AV nicking (A:V = 1:4)
   c. Flame hemorrhages
   d. Occasional soft, cotton-wool exudates
4. Grade IV
   a. Silver wire arterioles
   b. Marked AV nicking (A:V = 1:4)
   c. Flame hemorrhages
   d. Many soft exudates
   e. Hard, shiny macular exudates (star pattern)
   f. Papilledema

## HYPERTENSION: A SIMPLIFIED
## THERAPEUTIC APPROACH

Who should be treated? The Joint National Committee on Detection, Evaluation and Treatment of High Blood Pressure has made the following recommendations:

1. Diastolic pressure >120 mm Hg; treat immediately
2. Diastolic pressure 105–119; treat
3. Diastolic pressure 90–104; treat unless contraindicated

Current recommendations for treating systolic hypertension are

1. Age <35 years, treat systolic pressure >140 mm Hg
2. Age 35–59, treat systolic pressure >150
3. Age >60, treat systolic pressure >160

The goal of treatment is to return the diastolic pressure to 90 mm Hg, and to reduce the systolic pressure by approximately 10% of its current value.

### Therapy

Where patient motivation and compliance are strong, and where blood pressure is only mildly elevated, great benefit can be gained through a program of salt restriction, weight loss, increased physical activity and relaxation.

Even while pursuing the above modalities, most patients will require some pharmacologic intervention. Initially this will usually be a thiazide diuretic and/or a $\beta$-blocker (propranolol or a specific $\beta_1$ agent, such as metoprolol).

| *Thiazide Preferred In* | *β-Blocker Preferred In* |
|---|---|
| Elderly patients* | Young patients |
| Patients with low plasma renins | Patients with evidence of autonomic overactivity |
| | Patients with labile hypertension |
| | Patients with high plasma renins |

*Many elderly patients require a combination of a thiazide diuretic with either a potassium-sparing diuretic or KCL supplementation.

## HYPERTENSION: A SIMPLIFIED
## THERAPEUTIC APPROACH *(cont.)*

If control is inadequate within 1–2 months, combine the diuretic with propranolol or another sympatholytic agent, such as methyldopa or clonidine.

If control is still inadequate notwithstanding increasing doses of drugs, the patient has severe disease and several options can be tried:

1. Add hydralazine to the diuretic and sympatholytic
2. Continue the diuretic and substitute guanethidine or clonidine for the sympatholytic
3. Combine two sympatholytics that act in different ways (e.g., propranolol and prazosin)

## ANTIHYPERTENSIVE DRUGS

| Drug | Mechanism of Action | Principal Side Effects | Comments |
|---|---|---|---|
| *Diuretics* | | | |
| *Thiazides* | | | |
| Chlorthiazide (Diuril), Hydrochlorthiazide (Hydro-Diuril) | Inhibit Na⁺ resorption in distal tubule | Hypokalemia, hyperglycemia, hyperuricemia, hypercalcemia | May precipitate gouty arthritis |
| *Phthalimidines* | | | |
| Chlorthalidone (Hygroton) Metolazone (Zaroxolyn) | | | |
| *Loop diuretics* | | | |
| Furosemide (Lasix) Ethacrynic acid (Edecrin) | Inhibit Na⁺ resorption in loop of Henle | Profound hypokalemia and metabolic alkalosis, hyperuricemia, GI distress, eighth nerve damage | Because of the danger of severe electrolyte imbalances, thiazides are generally preferred |
| *Potassium sparers* | | | |
| Spironolactone (Aldactone) Triamterene (Dyrenium) | Spironolactone is an aldosterone antagonist; triamterene directly affects tubular transport | Hyperkalemia, GI distress, fatigue, gynecomastia | Often combined with thiazides because of opposing effects on potassium secretion |

## ANTIHYPERTENSIVE DRUGS *(cont.)*

### *Vasodilators*

| | | | |
|---|---|---|---|
| Hydralazine (Apresoline) Minoxidil (Loniten) Nitroprusside (Nipride) Diazoxide (Hyperstat) | Relax arteriolar smooth muscle and thus decrease peripheral resistance; nitroprusside relaxes both arteriolar and venous smooth muscle | Increased sympathetic activity (reflex tachycardia, increased myocardial work) and Na$^+$ retention. Hydralazine: SLE-like syndrome (dose and duration related), orthostatic hypotension. Minoxidil: hypertrichosis. Nitroprusside: cyanide poisoning (dose related), nausea, vomiting, substeral discomfort, sweating, anxiety. Diazoxide: hyperglycemia, sedation | Hydralazine and minoxidil are not used alone because the reflex sympathetic activity may cause angina or an MI; they are effective in combination with a $\beta$-blocker and a diuretic. Nitroprusside is an extremely powerful drug used (without reported failures) in hypertensive emergencies in ICU only |

### *Sympatholytics*

| | | | |
|---|---|---|---|
| Clonidine (Catapres) | Stimulates adrenergic receptors within the CNS, thus inhibiting peripheral sympathetic activity | Constipation, fluid retention, impotence, rebound hypertension | Impotence less common than with methyldopa |

| Methyldopa (Aldomet) | Acts within the CNS and may also suppress renin release | Sedation, depression, fluid retention, dry mouth, headache, dry fever, elevated hepatic enzymes, impotence, galactorrhea, hemolytic anemia | Twenty percent of patients become Coombs positive; contraindicated in patients with active liver disease |
| --- | --- | --- | --- |
| Reserpine (Serpasil) | Depletes the CNS store of catecholamines | Depression, bradycardia, GI cramps, diarrhea, increased appetite, fatigue | Contraindicated in patients with depressive disorders or peptic ulcer disease |

*Peripheral sympatholytics*

*β-Blockers*

| Propranolol (Inderal) Metoprolol (Lopressor) | β-Adrenergic receptor antagonists; metoprolol acts selectively on the heart ($\beta_1$ antagonist); propranolol suppresses central adrenergic activity, acts directly on heart and suppresses renin release | Propranolol; bradycardia, fatigue, nausea, diarrhea, bronchoconstriction Metoprolol; fatigue, dizziness, headache, insomnia, depression, diarrhea | Both drugs can mask the symptoms of hypoglycemia and should be used with caution in diabetics; they may also precipitate congestive heart failure and AV block; propranolol is contraindicated in patients with bronchial asthma |
| --- | --- | --- | --- |

## ANTIHYPERTENSIVE DRUGS *(cont.)*

*α-Blockers*

| | | | |
|---|---|---|---|
| Prazosin (Minipress) | Prazosin is a specific antagonist to the postsynaptic α-receptor | Fluid retention, drowsiness, orthostatic hypotension, headache, palpitations | Often combined with a diuretic or a β-blocker in patients with severe hypertension |

*Combined α- and β-blockers*

| | | | |
|---|---|---|---|
| Guanethidine (Ismelin) | Inhibit α- and β-adrenergic responses | Severe orthostatic hypotension, diarrhea, weakness, fluid retention, impotence, ejaculatory dysfunction | The frequency and severity of side effects have limited the use of guanethidine to severe hypertension which is refractory to other agents |

*Ganglionic blocking agents*

| | | | |
|---|---|---|---|
| Trimethaphan (Arfonad) | Blocks both sympathetic and parasympathetic activity by disrupting transmission in autonomic ganglia | Tachycardia, mydriasis, constipation, urinary retention, dry mouth, anhidrosis, anorexia, severe orthostatic hypotension | Effective in hypertension associated with an acute aortic dissection |

*Converting
enzyme inhibitor*

| | | | |
|---|---|---|---|
| Captopril (Capoten) | Prevents activation of renin—angiotensin—aldosterone mechanism | Fever, rash, granulocytopenia, stomatitis, proteinuria, glomerulonephritis, altered taste perception | May be extremely effective when all other drugs have failed, especially in patients with high renin levels |

# Section

# 2

# Pulmonary
# Disease

## ARTERIAL BLOOD GASES: NORMAL VALUES*

|                                   | *Arterial* | *Venous* |
|-----------------------------------|------------|----------|
| $O_2$ tension, mm Hg              | 93         | 40       |
| $CO_2$ tension, mm Hg             | 40         | 46       |
| Dissolved $O_2$, vol%             | 0.3        | 0.1      |
| Total $O_2$, vol%                 | 19.8       | 15.2     |
| $O_2$ capacity of Hb, vol%        | 20.1       | 20.1     |
| $O_2$ saturation of Hb, vol.%     | 97         | 75       |
| Hemoglobin, g per 100 ml          | 15         | 15       |
| Dissolved $CO_2$, vol%            | 2.5        | 2.9      |
| $CO_2$ content, vol%              | 46         | 50       |
| Plasma $CO_2$ content, vol%       | 56         | 60       |
| Plasma $CO_2$ content, mM         | 25         | 27       |
| Plasma pH                         | 7.38       | 7.35     |

*From CH Best, NB Taylor: The physiological basis of medical practice, 9th edition, Baltimore: Williams & Wilkins. © (1978) The Williams & Wilkins Co., Baltimore.

## ALTERATIONS IN HEMOGLOBIN AFFINITY FOR OXYGEN

By far the most important causes of tissue hypoxia are arterial hypoxemia (usually due to pulmonary disease) and reduced blood flow (either global—a reduction in cardiac output—or regional). A much less common cause of tissue hypoxia is an increased affinity of hemoglobin for oxygen, making oxygen delivery to the tissues more difficult. A decreased affinity for oxygen by itself usually causes no difficulty, but can, in combination with cardiopulmonary disease, compromise tissue oxygenation.

### Important Causes of Increased Affinity (Shift to the Left)

1. Acute alkalosis (Bohr effect)
2. Decreased $PCO_2$
3. Decreased 2,3-diphosphoglycerate
   a. Hypophosphatemia
   b. Transfusions with stored blood
   c. Chronic acidosis
   d. Red blood cell enzyme disorders
4. Hypothermia
5. Hemoglobinopathies
   a. Congenital
   b. Acquired
      i. Methemoglobin (caused by nitrites and other oxidants; can also be congenital)
      ii. Carboxyhemoglobin (carbon monoxide poisoning)

### Important Causes of Decreased Affinity (Shift to the Right)

1. Acute acidosis (Bohr effect)
2. Increased $PCO_2$
3. Increased 2,3-diphosphoglycerate
   a. Normal response to high altitude, anemia, cardiac or pulmonary disease, and blood loss
   b. Exercise adaptation
   c. Chronic alkalosis
   d. Red blood cell enzyme disorders
   e. Hyperphosphatemia
4. Hyperthermia
5. Hemoglobinopathies: congenital

# ALTERATIONS IN HEMOGLOBIN
# AFFINITY FOR OXYGEN *(cont.)*

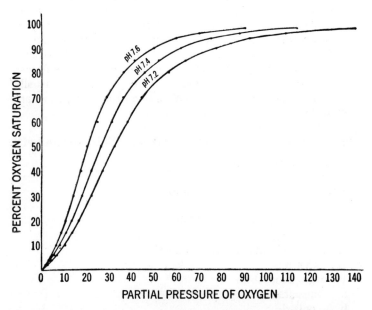

Oxygen dissociation curves of human hemoglobin at various pH values. (Harris, J.W. and Kellermeyer, R.W.: The Red Cell, Revised ed., Harvard University Press, Cambridge, Mass., 1970. Reprinted by permission.)

## CAUSES OF HYPERVENTILATION

1. Anxiety (hyperventilation syndrome), tension or pain
2. Metabolic acidosis
3. Drugs (most often salicylates and amphetamines)
4. Cerebrovascular accident
5. Shock
6. Fever
7. Anemia
8. Hyperthyroidism
9. Interstitial lung diseases
10. Pulmonary embolism

## CAUSES OF ACUTE RESPIRATORY FAILURE

1. Decompensation of chronic lung disease
2. Acute airway obstruction
    a. Epiglottitis
    b. Croup
    3. Aspiration of a foreign body
    d. Asthma
    e. Bronchiolitis
3. Viral and bacterial pneumonias
4. Pulmonary emboli
5. Pneumothorax
6. Chest trauma (fractured ribs, flail chest)
7. Cardiogenic pulmonary edema
8. Adult respiratory distress syndrome (ARDS; noncardiogenic pulmonary edema)
    a. Shock
    b. Infection
    c. Fat emboli
    d. Chest trauma
    e. Aspiration
    f. Pancreatitis
    g. Inhaled toxins (oxygen, smoke, chemicals)
    h. Drug overdose
    i. Burns
    j. Disseminated intravascular coagulation (DIC)
    k. Massive blood transfusion
    l. Postoperative (especially cardiopulmonary bypass)
    m. Fluid overload
    n. Near-fatal drowning
    o. Capillary leak syndrome (idiopathic)
9. Global alveolar hypoventilation
    a. Neuromuscular disorders
        i. CNS suppression from sedatives, analgesics, alcohol, etc.
        ii. Spinal cord injuries
        iii. Polyneuritis (e.g., Guillain-Barré syndrome)
        iv. Poliomyelitis
        v. Myasthenic crisis
    b. Severe hypothyroidism
    c. Severe metabolic alkalosis
    d. Sleep-apnea syndrome
    e. Pickwickian syndrome

## COMPLICATIONS OF INTUBATION AND MECHANICAL VENTILATION

1. Mechanical failure
2. Improper placement of tube in right main stem bronchus
3. Superinfection
4. Accumulation of secretions
5. Tracheal stenosis and tracheomalacia
6. Pneumothorax, pneumomediastinum, subcutaneous emphysema
7. Iatrogenic hyperventilation
8. Respiratory alkalosis
9. Cardiac arrhythmias
10. Atelectasis
11. Gastrointestinal bleeding
12. Pulmonary embolism
13. Oxygen toxicity
14. Psychological trauma
15. Complications of PEEP include
    a. Decreased venous return and cardiac output
    b. Gastric dilatation and rupture
    c. Syndrome of inappropriate ADH secretion

## CAUSES OF HEMOPTYSIS

1. Pulmonary infections
   a. Chronic bronchitis
   b. Bronchiectasis
   c. Pneumonia
   d. Tuberculosis
   e. Lung abscess
   f. Fungal infection (especially aspergillosis)
2. Pulmonary neoplasms
   a. Bronchogenic carcinoma
   b. Bronchial adenoma
3. Other pulmonary disorders
   a. AV malformations
   b. Trauma
   c. Aspiration of a foreign body
   d. Pulmonary hypertension
   e. Idiopathic pulmonary hemosiderosis
4. Cardiac disorders
   a. Mitral stenosis
   b. Pulmonary edema
5. Systemic disorders
   a. Pulmonary infarction (secondary to pulmonary embolism)
   b. Coagulation disorders
   c. Sarcoidosis
   d. Goodpasture's syndrome
   f. Osler-Weber-Rendu syndrome
   g. Wegener's granulomatosis

## THE DIAGNOSIS OF PULMONARY EMBOLI

### Symptoms (In Order of Decreasing Frequency)

1. More than 50% of patients
   a. Dyspnea
   b. Pleuritic chest pain
   c. Anxiety and restlessness
   d. Nonproductive cough
2. Fewer than 50% of patients
   a. Hemoptysis
   b. Sweating
   c. Syncope
   d. Anginalike chest pain (only with massive emboli)

### Signs (In Order of Decreasing Frequency)

1. More than 50% of patients
   a. Tachypnea
   b. Rales
   c. Increased pulmonic valve closure sound
2. Fewer than 50% of patients
   a. Tachycardia
   b. Fever
   c. Thrombophlebitis
   d. $S_3$ or $S_4$ gallop
   e. Diaphoresis
   f. Pleural friction rub
   g. Cyanosis
   h. Arrhythmias
   i. Wheezing
   j. Shock

### Chest X-ray (The Most Common Findings)

1. Parenchymal infiltrate (45–55%)
2. Diaphragmatic elevation (40–45%)
3. Pleural effusion (35–50%)
4. Prominent pulmonary vessels (15–40%)

## THE DIAGNOSIS OF PULMONARY EMBOLI *(cont.)*

### ECG

1. Tachycardia
2. ST and T wave abnormalities
3. P pulmonale
4. Right ventricular strain

### Laboratory and Diagnostic Tests

1. Elevated LDH (80%)
2. Triad of elevated LDH, elevated bilirubin, and normal SGOT in only 5–12% of patients
3. Elevated fibrin split products
4. White blood cell count rarely exceeds 15,000
5. Perfusion scan: no perfusion
6. Ventilation scan: normal (unless there is infarction)
7. Angiography is the definitive test. Either of two findings is virtually diagnostic: (1) complete vessel cutoff, and (2) a filling defect within a vessel.

# PLEURAL EFFUSIONS

## Symptoms

1. Often asymptomatic.
2. If the effusion is large or accumulates rapidly, the most common complaints are dyspnea, cough, and pleuritic chest pain.

## Examination

1. Small effusions (<500 ml) usually produce no findings on physical examination. Chest x-ray may reveal blunting of the costophrenic angles on lateral and decubitus films.
2. Larger effusions may be accompanied by diminished fremitus and breath sounds, dullness to percussion and rales over adjacent pulmonary parenchyma. Chest x-ray may reveal a large opacity, the upper margin of which forms a meniscus along the lateral wall. A mediastinal shift may also be seen.

## Differential Diagnosis

1. The key to diagnosing the cause of an effusion lies in determining whether the effusion is a *transudate* (low in protein) or an *exudate* (high in protein). This requires a *diagnostic thoracentesis.*
2. If the following three criteria are met, the effusion is almost certainly an exudate:
   a. The ratio of total protein in the effusion to total protein in the serum is greater than 0.5.
   b. The concentration of LDH in the effusion is greater than 200 IU/L.
   c. The ratio of LDH in the effusion to LDH in the serum is greater than 0.6.

## Mechanism of Formation

1. Transudates are generally caused by imbalances in the Starling forces governing formation and resorption of pleural fluid.
2. Exudates are generally the result of inflammation and malignancy.

## Causes of Transudates

1. Congestive heart failure.
2. Cirrhosis.
3. Nephrotic syndrome.
4. Meig's syndrome.

## PLEURAL EFFUSIONS *(cont.)*

5. Superior vena caval obstruction.
6. Malignancy (much more often an exudate).
7. Myxedema.
8. Peritoneal dialysis.
9. Hypoalbuminemia due to malabsorption.

### Causes of Exudates

1. Malignancy (primary lung cancer—especially adenocarcinoma; also metastatic cancer, leukemia, lymphoma, pleural mesothelioma).
2. Infection (especially bacterial pneumonia and tuberculosis, but any pulmonary infection can be responsible).
3. Pulmonary embolism with infarction.
4. Asbestosis.
5. Trauma.
6. Pneumothorax.
7. Chylothorax.
8. Sarcoidosis (very rarely associated with an effusion).
9. Pancreatitis.
10. Subphrenic abscess.
11. Esophageal rupture.
12. Connective tissue diseases (most often SLE or rheumatoid arthritis).
13. Dressler's syndrome.
14. Uremia.

### Special Notes

1. Grossly hemorrhagic effusions are most commonly seen with malignancy, infarction, and trauma, and occasionally with pancreatitis.
2. Empyema is almost always associated with an underlying pneumonia, and is most often due to anaerobic infection (frequently following aspiration pneumonia), gram negative organisms (*E. coli*, *Klebsiella*, *Pseudomonas*, and *Enterobacter* predominate) or staphylococcus.
3. A low pleural fluid complement level can be seen in SLE and rheumatoid arthritis.
4. A high pleural fluid amylase can be seen in pancreatitis, ruptured esophagus, and malignancy.

## INFECTIOUS MONONUCLEOSIS

### Symptoms

1. Common (>50% of patients)
   a. Sore throat
   b. Malaise
   c. Fatigue
   d. Headache
2. Less common
   a. Chills
   b. Myalgias
   c. Arthralgias
   d. Anorexia
   e. GI discomfort with nausea and vomiting

### Signs

1. Common (>50% of patients)
   a. Cervical lymphadenopathy
   b. Mild fever
   c. Splenomegaly
2. Less common
   a. Generalized lymphadenopathy
   b. Hepatomegaly
   c. Palatal petechiae
   d. Transient macular rash on trunk
   e. Periorbital edema
   f. Jaundice

### Rare Complications (<1% of patients)

1. Splenic rupture
2. CNS involvement (meningitis, encephalitis, Guillain-Barré; Bell's palsy)
3. Hemolytic anemia
4. Thrombocytopenic purpura
5. Pericarditis
6. Myocarditis

## INFECTIOUS MONONUCLEOSIS *(cont.)*

**Laboratory Findings**

1. Increased liver function tests
2. Atypical lymphocytosis
3. Increased antibody titers to the Ebstein-Barr virus
4. High titers of heterophil antibody (an IgM antibody that agglutinates sheep red blood cells)
5. False positive tests for syphilis and rheumatoid factor
6. Red cells become Coombs positive

## VIRAL AND MYCOPLASMAL PNEUMONIA: DIFFERENTIATING FEATURES

### Viral Pneumonia

1. *Etiologic agent:* typically influenza virus or adenovirus
2. *Spread:* highly contagious, occurs in community epidemics
3. *Incubation:* 1–3 days
4. *Onset:* may be gradual or acute, with fever, headache, myalgias, weakness, rhinorrhea and pharyngitis; rigors are unusual, although a single episode may sometimes occur with influenza
5. *Pneumonic manifestations:* cough and dyspnea herald the development of pneumonia 1–3 days after the prodrome; pleuritic chest pain is rare
6. *Physical exam:* dry rales
7. *Sputum:* cough is initially nonproductive, but, later, sputum may become thick with leucocytes and epithelial cells
8. *Chest x-ray:* bilateral fluffy infiltrates, effusions may be present, consolidation is rare
9. *Duration:* typically 1–2 weeks

### Mycoplasmal pneumonia

1. *Etiologic agent: Mycoplasma pneumoniae*
2. *Spread:* not highly contagious, limited to close contacts (family, school, etc.); generally limited to persons 5–30 years old.
3. *Incubation:* 1–5 weeks
4. *Onset:* very gradual with fever, myalgias, coryza, and pharyngitis
5. *Pneumonic manifestations:* pneumonia develops slowly, with cough, pleuritic chest pain in 20%, and bullous myringitis in 10–15%; some patients develop skin rashes
6. *Physical exam:* dry rales
7. *Sputum:* nonproductive cough may give way to sputum containing leucocytes without bacteria
8. *Chest x-ray:* diffuse infiltrates with predilection for lower lobes; effusions in 20%; consolidation is rare
9. *Duration:* typically 2–6 weeks

## INFLUENZA WITH SECONDARY
## BACTERIAL PNEUMONIA

The development of a bacterial pneumonia following an influenza infection as opposed to a simple influenza pneumonia can usually be recognized as follows:

1. Acute clinical deterioration several days after the influenza prodrome, unlike the rapid, uninterrupted progression of influenza pneumonia
2. Production of purulent sputum containing bacteria and leukocytes
3. A high white blood cell count (greater than 15,000)
4. An elevated ESR
5. The chest x-ray may reveal focal consolidation or even cavitation

## BACTERIAL PNEUMONIAS

| Organism | Typical chest x-ray features | Typical appearance of sputum | Comments |
|---|---|---|---|
| *Pneumococcus* | Dense, homogeneous consolidation with air bronchograms; only one lobe (often lower or middle) may be involved; cavitation is rare; effusions in 10–15% of cases. | Rust-colored during peak of illness | Most common bacterial pneumonia, especially in otherwise healthy persons; often a preceding UTI; herpes labialis is present in 40% of cases. |
| *Staphylococcus aureus* | Patchy, widespread infiltration with many rounded areas of consolidation; very rapid spread and cavitation; pneumatoceles develop in children, rarely in adults; majority develop effusions. | Pink or blood-streaked | Commonly seen post-influenza and in patients with diminished resistence to infection; may see staphylococcal skin lesions; empyema in 10% of cases; high mortality. |
| *Streptococcus pyogenes* | Patchy bronchopneumonia; consolidation and cavity formation are rare; majority develop effusions. | Thin, pink | Very rare, except as a complication of a preceding respiratory infection and in epidemics among army recruits; key feature is early development of empyema in approx. 50%; 10–15% develop bacteremia. |
| *Hemophilus influenzae* | Patchy bronchopneumonia, less often a lobar pneumonia; cavitation is rare; effusions in one third of cases. | Thick, apple-green | Mostly seen in children; in adults, usually seen in alcholics and patients with chronic lung disease |

## BACTERIAL PNEUMONIAS *(cont.)*

| | | | |
|---|---|---|---|
| *Klebsiella pneumoniae* (Friedlander's bacillus) | Dense lobar consolidation with air bronchograms; several lobes, especially the upper lobes, may be involved; swollen parenchyma with bulging fissures is often seen (*before* cavitation, unlike other pneumonias); early cavitation; effusions are common | Thick, red-brown ("current jelly") sputum | Seen in debilitated patients, especially alchoholics; bacteremia is common—20% develop jaundice; high mortality |
| *Escherichia coli* | Bronchopneumonia involving the lower lobes; effusions are common; cavity formation is rare. | Thick | In debilitated patients, often results from spread from GI or renal infection; empyema in 40% of cases; high mortality. |
| *Pseudomonas aeruginosa* | Diffuse nodular bronchopneumonia involving the lower lobes; early cavitation. | Copious yellow or green | In debilitated patients, often due to aspiration; 80% mortality. |
| *Legionnella pneumophila* (Legionnaire's Disease) | Patchy bronchopneumoria progressing to consolidation; rapid involvement of entire lobe and lung; small effusions in 30–40%. | Scanty, non-purulent | A severe, rapidly progressive disease with systemic symptoms (myalgias, GI distress, encephalopathy). |

## BACTERIAL PNEUMONIA:
## SOME AIDS IN DIAGNOSIS

1. A properly obtained sputum sample, acquired by deep coughing or transtracheal aspiration, is essential for diagnosing the cause of acute pneumonia. The presence of squamous epithelial cells in the sample indicates that the sputum did not come from deep enough in the lung, since these cells are found in the mouth.
2. Pneumococcus and hemophilus can be difficult to grow from sputum cultures. In addition, at least 25% of healthy individuals carry pneumococcus in their upper respiratory tract, and over 50% carry hemophilus. Other normal flora that may complicate the diagnosis include streptococci (almost everyone carries some streptococcus species, although uncommonly streptococcus pyogenes) and, less often, gram negative aerobes.
3. Sputum cultures take 2-3 days to grow and should be supplemented with blood cultures. In most cases of hemophilus pneumonia the organism can be grown from the blood.
4. The major causes of pneumonia following an episode of influenza are
   a. *Staphylococcus aureus*
   b. *Pneumococcus*
   c. *Hemophilus influenza*
5. The etiologic organism in aspiration pneumonias is largely determined by the setting in which it occurs:
   a. In the community: anaerobes (the predominant normal flora of the upper respiratory tract)
      i. *Bacteriodes melaninogenicus*
      ii. *Bacteroides fragilis*
      iii. *Fusobacterium*
      iv. *Peptostreptococcus*
   b. In the hospital: aerobes (or a mixture of aerobes and anaerobes)
      i. *Staphylococcus aureus*
      ii. *Enterobacteriaceae*
      iii. *Pseudomonas*
6. Aspiration occurs most often with the patient supine, and pneumonia typically develops in the dependent areas of the lungs:
   a. The superior segments of the lower lobes
   b. The superior segment of the left upper lobe
   c. The posterior segment of the right upper lobe

## PRIMARY DRUGS IN THE
## TREATMENT OF TUBERCULOSIS

1. Isoniazid (INH)
   a. Administration: oral
   b. Metabolism: acetylated in the liver, excreted by the kidney
   c. CSF penetration: yes
   d. Side effects: hepatitis (increased risk in rapid acetylators) and neuritis (peripheral neuropathy and CNS involvement, including seizures and psychosis)
   e. Monitor toxicity: liver function tests
   f. Drug interactions
      i. Interferes with metabolism of phenytoin
      ii. Increased risk of hepatotoxicity when combined with rifampin
   g. Comments: neurotoxicity can be prevented with daily pyridoxine
2. Ethambutol
   a. Administration: oral
   b. Metabolism: excreted, mostly unchanged, by the kidney
   c. CSF penetration: no, although may penetrate with meningitis
   d. Side effects: optic neuritis (diminished visual acuity and red-green color discrimination)
   e. Monitor toxicity: opthalmologic examinations
   f. Comments: optic neuritis is generally reversible if drug is discontinued
3. Streptomycin
   a. Administration: intramuscular
   b. Metabolism: excreted, mostly unchanged, by the kidney
   c. CSF penetration: no
   d. Side effects: eighth nerve damage (especially the vestibular portion), renal toxicity, hypersensitivity reactions
   e. Monitor toxicity: audiograms, BUN, and creatinine
4. Rifampin
   a. Administration: oral
   b. Metabolism: metabolized in liver, most is excreted in bile but some metabolites appear in the urine, coloring it orange
   c. CSF penetration: yes
   d. Side effects: hepatotoxicity, thrombocytopenia, hypersensitivity reactions, flulike syndrome
   e. Monitor toxicity: liver function tests
   f. Drug interactions: increases metabolism of birth control pills and anticoagulants

## CAUSES OF WHEEZING

1. Pulmonary
   a. Aspiration of a foreign body
   b. Tracheal stenosis
   c. Laryngeal stridor
   d. Asthma
   e. COPD
   f. Pulmonary embolism
   g. Tumors and granulomas impinging on the main airways
2. Nonpulmonary
   a. Cardiac asthma
   b. Anaphylaxis
   c. Carcinoid syndrome
   d. Allergic angiitis

## ALLERGIC VS. NONALLERGIC ASTHMA

|  | *Allergic* | *Nonallergic* |
|---|---|---|
| Pathophysiology | Sensitized mast cells release bronchoconstricting substances (histamine, SRS-A) | Irritant submucous receptors trigger vagal reflexes |
| Onset | Childhood, early adulthood | Adulthood |
| Family history of atopy | Positive | Negative |
| Skin tests to specific allergens | Positive | Negative |
| Serum IgE levels | High in >50% | Normal |
| Other allergies | Common | Uncommon |
| Course | Seasonal | Continual |
| Status asthmaticus | Less common | More common |

## CAUSES OF HYPERSENSITIVITY PNEUMONITIS (EXTRINSIC ALLERGIC ALVEOLITIS)

| Disease | Contact with antigen | Antigen |
|---|---|---|
| Paper mill-worker's lung | Moldy wood pulp | *Alternaria* |
| Woodworker's lung | Wood dust, moldy logs | *Alternaria* |
| Malt worker's lung | Moldy barley or malt dust | *Aspergillus fumigatus, Aspergillus clavatus* |
| Maple bark-stripper's lung | Moldy maple bark | *Cryptostroma corticale* |
| Sequoiosis | Redwood sawdust | *Graphium* |
| Paprika splitter's lung | Paprika dust | *Mucor stolonifer* |
| Cheese worker's lung | Moldy cheese | *Penicillium frequetans* |
| Wheat-weevil lung | Infested wheat flour | *Sitophilus granarius* |
| Farmer's lung | Moldy hay or grain | Thermophilic actinomycetes, *Micropolyspora faeni* |
| Bagassosis | Moldy sugar cane | Thermophilic actinomycetes |
| Air-conditioner or humidifier lung | Contaminated water | Thermophilic actinomycetes |
| Mushroom worker's lung | Mushroom compost | Thermophilic actinomycetes |
| Bird fancier's lung | Droppings and feathers of pigeons, parakeets, chickens, and turkeys | Unknown |

## CAUSES OF HYPERSENSITIVITY PNEUMONITIS (EXTRINSIC ALLERGIC ALVEOLITIS) *(cont.)*

| Disease | Source of antigen | Antigen |
|---------|-------------------|---------|
| Coffee worker's lung | Coffee bean dust | Unknown |
| Furrier's lung | Animal fur dust | Unknown |
| Pituitary snuff-taker's lung | Pituitary extracts | Unknown |
| Fishmeal worker's lung | Fishmeal dust | Unknown |

# CHRONIC OBSTRUCTIVE PULMONARY DISEASE: EMPHYSEMA VS. CHRONIC BRONCHITIS

| Features | Emphysema | Chronic Bronchitis |
|---|---|---|
| Pathophysiology | Loss of both air spaces and vasculature causes only minimal ventilation-perfusion mismatch | Fibrosis and mucous plugging of airways causes ventilation-perfusion mismatch that may be severe |

*Clinical manifestations*

| | | |
|---|---|---|
| General appearance | Thin, rosy-cheeked; "pink puffer" | Overweight, bull neck; "blue bloater" |
| Initial complaint | Dyspnea | Cough |
| Sputum production | Scant | Copious, often purulent |
| Cyanosis | Absent | Present |

*Physical exam*

| | | |
|---|---|---|
| Percussion | Hyperresonant | Normal |
| Auscultation | Decreased breath sounds | Rales and rhonchi |

| Chest x-ray | Low, flat diaphragms | Diaphragms are normal |
|---|---|---|
| | Lungs are hyperlucent | Lungs are normal or fibrotic |
| | Heart is small | Heart is large |

*Laboratory*

| | | |
|---|---|---|
| Arterial $P_{O_2}$ | Slightly decreased | May be severely decreased |
| Arterial $P_{CO_2}$ | Rises terminally | Early and progressive elevation |
| Red cell mass | Normal | Increased |
| Total lung capacity | Increased | Normal or slightly increased |
| FEV1 and VC | Decreased | Decreased |

## CHRONIC OBSTRUCTIVE PULMONARY DISEASE: EMPHYSEMA VS. CHRONIC BRONCHITIS *(cont.)*

| *Features* | *Emphysema* | *Chronic Bronchitis* |
|---|---|---|
| Residual volume | Increased | Increased |
| Lung compliance | Increased | Normal |
| Diffusing capacity | Decreased | Normal or decreased |

| *Complications* | | |
|---|---|---|
| Cor pulmonale and pulmonary hypertension | Terminally, and occasionally during bouts of infection | Early in course |
| Recurrent infections | Occasional; may precipitate terminal decline | Often; contribute to progressive downhill course |

## LUNG CANCER: CLINICAL MANIFESTATIONS

| *Manifestation* | *Comments* |
|---|---|

*Pulmonary involvement*

| | |
|---|---|
| 1. Cough | Most common presenting symptom |
| 2. Sputum production | — |
| 3. Dyspnea | — |
| 4. Hemoptysis | Usually only blood-tinged sputum |
| 5. Wheezing | Only if airway is compressed |
| 6. Infection | Suspect an underlying malignancy in a patient with pneumonia when |
| | 1. Response to antibiotics is prolonged |
| | 2. X-ray clearing is incomplete |
| | 3. Infection recurs in the same location |

*Local spread*

| | |
|---|---|
| 1. Chest pain | Typically pleuritic, but may also be due to chest wall invasion |
| 2. Hoarseness | Due to involvement of the recurrent laryngeal nerve, usually on the left side (where the nerve has a longer course) |
| 3. Pancoast syndrome | Apical tumors may impinge on the brachial plexus (causing pain in the shoulder or arm) and the inferior cervical sympathetic ganglion (producing Horner's syndrome with ipsilateral partial eyelid ptosis, pupillary constriction, enopthalmos, and warmth and dryness on the face) |
| 4. Superior vena caval obstruction | Suffusion, edema, and cyanosis of face, neck, and arms (first sign may be inability to button shirts due to neck enlargement), headache and dizziness worsened by bending forward, varicosities on chest wall and shoulders |
| 5. Dysphagia | Due to esophageal compression |

*Metastases*

| | |
|---|---|
| 1. Lymphadenopathy | Especially cervical and supraclavicular |
| 2. Bone involvement | Bone pain |
| 3. Liver involvement | Jaundice, abdominal discomfort |
| 4. CNS involvement | Symptoms may be many and varied |
| 5. Adrenal involvement | Rarely symptomatic |

*Systemic manifestations*

| | |
|---|---|
| 1. Clubbing | Associated with a great many diseases and thus of little help in diagnosis |

## LUNG CANCER: CLINICAL MANIFESTATIONS *(cont.)*

| *Manifestation* | *Comments* |
|---|---|
| 2. Hypertrophic osteoarthropathy | Swelling, pain, and tenderness over distal long bones; usually seen with tumors involving the pleura |
| 3. Dermatomyositis | — |
| 4. Acanthosis nigricans | Dark, velvety skin lesions in the body folds; much more commonly seen with GI malignancies |

*Endocrine disorders*

| | |
|---|---|
| 1. Hyperparathyroidism | Ectopic hormone production by the tumor Hypercalcemia may also be due to bone metastases |
| 2. Syndrome of inappropriate ADH secretion | Seen with oat cell tumors |
| 3. Gynecomastia | — |
| 4. Cushing's syndrome | — |
| 5. Carcinoid syndrome | — |

*Neuromuscular disorders*

| | |
|---|---|
| 1. Weakness | Common; usually proximal |
| 2. Eaton-Lambert syndrome | Weakness of pelvic and limb musculature; a disorder of the neuromuscular junction but, unlike myasthenia gravis, spares the ocular musculature and improves with repeated stimulation |
| 3. Peripheral neuropathy | May be sensory, motor, or mixed |
| 4. Cerebellar degeneration | Very rare |

*Vascular and hematologic disorders*

| | |
|---|---|
| 1. Thrombophlebitis | — |
| 2. Nonbacterial thrombotic endocarditis | — |
| 3. Chronic anemia | — |
| 4. Hemolytic anemia | — |
| 5. Thrombocytopenic purpura | — |
| 6. Cryofibrinoginemia | — |

## DIFFERENTIAL DIAGNOSIS OF THE
## SOLITARY PULMONARY NODULE

### Causes

1. Neoplasms (< 25%)
   a. Bronchogenic carcinoma
   b. Bronchial adenoma
   c. Lung metastases
2. Benign lesions (> 75%)
   a. Granulomas (approximately 60% of cases; usually tuberculosis of fungi)
   b. Hamartoma (a benign connective tissue tumor)
   c. Bronchogenic cyst
   d. Circumscribed pneumonia
   e. Very rare causes:
      i. Rheumatoid granuloma
      ii. Hydatid cyst
      iii. AV fistula
      iv. Abscess
      v. Hematoma
      vi. Wegener's granulomatosis
      vii. Pulmonary infarct (rarely appears as a solitary nodule)
3. High suspicion of malignancy in patients
   a. Who are over 40 years of age,
   b. Who smoke
   c. Whose chest x-ray features suggest possible malignancy

### X-ray Features of Solitary Pulmonary Nodules

4. *Most reliable—Calcification*
   a. If tomography reveals calcification within the nodule, it is most likely benign (the major exception—ossifying metastases of osteogenic sarcoma)
5. *Fairly reliable—Rate of growth*
   a. If the nodule has persisted unchanged for more than 2 years, it is probably benign
   b. If the nodule has doubled in size in one month, it is probably an inflammatory lesion and benign
   c. Any nodule showing an intermediate rate of growth must be highly suspected of malignancy

## DIFFERENTIAL DIAGNOSIS OF THE
## SOLITARY PULMONARY NODULE *(cont.)*

6. *Less reliable*
   a. Fuzziness or irregularity of the nodule border suggests malignancy
   b. Notching or umbilication of the nodule border suggests malignancy
7. Surgical resection of a solitary nodule is indicated unless
   a. Initial evaluation has proven the nodule benign beyond reasonable doubt
   b. The tumor has already metastasized
   c. Surgery would be too risky for the patient

## DISORDERS ASSOCIATED WITH
## SYMMETRICAL CLUBBING

1. *Pulmonary*
   a. Lung cancer (primary or metastatic)
   b. Interstitial fibrosis
   c. Cystic fibrosis
   d. Chronic infection (tuberculosis, empyema, abscess, bronchiectasis)
   e. AV malformations
   f. Chronic obstructive pulmonary disease
   g. Mesothelioma (tumors of the pleura)
   h. Lymphoma
2. *Cardiac*
   a. Infectious endocarditis
   b. Congenital heart disease with AV shunts
3. *Hyperthyroidism*
4. *Gastrointestinal*
   a. Hepatic cirrhosis
   b. Biliary cirrhosis
   c. Inflammatory bowel disease
   d. Neoplasms of the small and large intestine
   e. Malabsorption
5. Familial

## SARCOIDOSIS: CLINICAL MANIFESTATIONS

1. Pulmonary complaints: Fifty percent of patients present with one or several respiratory complaints:
   a. Dyspnea (the most common initial complaint)
   b. Nonproductive cough
   c. Chest pain (a vague discomfort, rarely pleuritic)
   d. Hemoptysis
   e. Pleural involvement (effusions are rare)
   f. Nasopharyngitis
2. Chest x-ray: Fifteen to twenty percent of patients are asymptomatic and are first diagnosed by an incidental finding on chest x-ray. Ninety percent of all patients will have an abnormal chest x-ray on presentation. Classic patterns include bilateral hilar adenopathy with or without parenchymal involvement, parenchymal involvement alone, and advanced fibrosis with bullae.
3. Constitutional complaints: Twenty-five percent of patients present with nonspecific constitutional complaints.
   a. Malaise
   b. Anorexia
   c. Weight loss
   d. Fever
4. *Extrapulmonary manifestations:* Five to ten percent of patients present with one of the less common extrathoracic manifestations.
   a. Dermatologic
      i. Erythema nodosum (usually bodes well for a mild, limited course)
      ii. Lupus pernio
      iii. Maculopapular lesions
      iv. Nodules
   b. Ocular
      i. Anterior uveitis (with watering, photophobia, pain, and diminished visual acuity)
      ii. Sjögren's syndrome
      iii. Retinopathy
      iv. Chorioretinitis
      v. Papilledema

    c. Cardiac
       i. Cor pulmonale
      ii. Cardiomyopathy
     iii. Heart block
     iv. Arrhythmias
    d. Renal
       i. Nephrocalcinosis
      ii. Nephrolithiasis
    e. Neurologic
       i. Cranial nerve palsies
      ii. Peripheral neuropathies
     iii. Basilar meningitis
     iv. Intracranial space-occupying lesions
      v. Spinal cord infiltration
    f. Other
       i. Hepatomegaly
      ii. Splenomegaly
     iii. Lymphadenopathy
     iv. Polyarthralgias and arthritis
      v. Myalgias and myopathy

5. *Laboratory*
    a. Hypercalciuria (often without hypercalcemia) is the most characteristic laboratory abnormality.
    b. Other findings may include elevated liver function tests, elevated serum uric acid, eosinophilia, an elevated ESR, occasionally a decreased red blood cell and white blood cell count.
    c. Immunologic abnormalities include hypergammaglobulinemia, diminished delayed hypersensitivity (skin test anergy), and a positive Kveim test.
    d. Angiotensin-converting enzyme frequently is elevated.

# Section

# 3

# Endocrinology

## THE HYPOTHALAMIC–PITUITARY AXIS

1. *Hypothalamic releasing factors*
   a. Stimulatory
      i. Thyrotropin releasing hormone (TRH)—effect is to stimulate release of TSH and prolactin
      ii. Growth hormone releasing factor (GHRF)—effect is to stimulate release of growth hormone
      iii. Gonadotropin (or luteinizing) releasing hormone (GnRH or LHRH)—effect is to stimulate release of LH and FSH
      iv. Corticotropin releasing factor (CRF)—effect is to stimulate release of ACTH
      v. (?) Prolactin releasing factor (PRF)—effect is to stimulate release of prolactin
      iv. (?) Melanocyte stimulating hormone releasing factor (MRF)—effect is to stimulate release of MSH
   Inhibitory
      i. Somatostatin (GHRIF)—effect is to inhibit release of growth hormone
      ii. Prolactin inhibiting factor (PIF)—effect is to inhibit release of prolactin
2. *Hormones of the anterior pituitary*
   a. Thyroid stimulating hormone (TSH)
      i. Excess: hyperthyroidism
      ii. Deficiency: hypothyroidism
   b. c. Luteinizing hormone (LH) and follicle-stimulating hormone (FSH)
      i. Excess:—
      ii. Deficiency: in adults, loss of libido, loss of pubic and axillary hair, atrophy of sexual organs, and may contribute to the development of the fine, wrinkled skin seen in panhypopituitarism
   d. Prolactin (PRL)
      i. Excess: in women, galactorrhea–amenorrhea syndrome; in men, infertility and impotence
      ii. Deficiency: in women, failure of lactation

    e. Growth hormone (GH)
      i. Excess: in adults, acromegaly
      ii. Deficiency: (?) hypoglycemia, and may also contribute to the dermatologic findings of panhypopituitarism
    f. Corticotropin (ACTH)
      i. Excess: Cushing's syndrome
      ii. Deficiency: adrenal cortical insufficiency
    g. Melanocyte-stimulating hormone (MSH)
      i. Excess: hyperpigmentation
      ii. Deficiency:—
3. *Hormones of the posterior pituitary*
    a. Vasopressin (ADH)
      i. Excess: syndrome of inappropriate ADH secretion (SIADH)
      ii. Deficiency: diabetes insipidus
    b. Oxytocin
      i. Deficiency in women, loss of milk-ejection reflex

## CAUSES OF HYPOPITUITARISM

Hypopituitarism is almost always synonymous with panhypopituitarism, since monotropic deficiencies are rare. Presenting features may include headache, visual disturbances (especially bitemporal hemianopid) and endocrine deficiencies. Gonadotropin and growth hormone are usually lost before TSH and ACTH, and thus if a man is potent and a woman cycling, the diagnosis of hypopituitarism should be reconsidered.

1. Neoplastic disease
    a. Tumors (usually a pituitary adenoma or a craniopharyngioma)
    b. Metastatic disease (especially lung and breast)
2. Iatrogenic
    a. Hypophysectomy
    b. Irradiation
3. Infection
    a. Tuberculosis
    b. Meningitis
    c. Encephalitis
4. Granulomatous diseases
    a. Sarcoidosis
    b. Histiocytosis X
5. Hemorrhage and Infarction
    a. Postpartum pituitary necrosis
    b. Trauma
    c. Cranial arteritis
    d. Sickle cell anemia
    e. Diabetes mellitus
    f. Cerebral aneurysms
    g. Vascular malformations
6. Hemochromatosis
7. Cysts
8. Idiopathic
9. Empty sella syndrome (only rarely do these patients have symptoms of pituitary hypofunction)

## ACROMEGALY: SIGNS AND SYMPTOMS

1. Local (parasellar) manifestations
   a. Common (>50%)
      i. Enlarged sella
      ii. Headache
      iii. Visual impairment
   b. Uncommon (<50%)
      i. Rhinorrhea
      ii. Uncinate seizures
      iii. Pituitary apoplexy
      iv. Papilledema
2. Systemic manifestations of increased growth hormone
   a. Common (>50%)
      i. Increased skeletal growth
      ii. Increased subcutaneous tissue growth
      iii. Hypermetabolism
      iv. Hyperhidrosis
      v. Arthralgias and arthritis
      vi. Hypertrichosis
      vii. Organomegaly
      viii. Deep voice
      ix. Osteoporosis
      x. Easy fatiguability and weakness
   b. Uncommon (<50%)
      i. Goiter
      ii. Hypertension
      iii. Glucose intolerance and frank diabetes mellitus
      iv. Decreased libido (males)
      v. Altered menses or amenorrhea
      vi. Gynecomastia
      vii. Galactorrhea
      viii. Cardiomyopathy
      ix. Auditory defects
      x. Hyperpigmentation
      xi. Fibroma molluscum
3. Laboratory findings
   a. Elevated growth hormone levels, not suppressed by glucose ingestion or other inhibitory stimuli (100%)
   b. Hypercalciuria (50%)
   c. Glycosuria (25%)
   d. Hyperprolactinemia (30%)

## CAUSES OF INAPPROPRIATE ANTIDIURETIC HORMONE SECRETION (SIADH)

1. Ectopic production of ADH
   a. Lung carcinoma (especially oat cell)
   b. Pancreatic carcinoma
   c. Duodenal carcinoma
   d. Hodgkin's disease
   e. Non-Hodgkin's lymphoma
   f. Thymoma
2. CNS disease
   a. Trauma
   b. Infection
   c. Stroke
   d. Brain tumors
   e. Seizure disorders
   f. Guillain-Barre syndrome
3. Pulmonary disease
   a. Tuberculosis
   b. Viral, bacterial, and fungal infection
4. Metabolic disease
   a. Myxedema
   b. Addison's disease
   c. Acute intermittent porphyria
5. Drugs
   a. Oxytocin
   b. Vasopressin
   c. Chlorpropamide
   d. Clofibrate
   e. Vincristine
   f. Vinblastine
   g. Cyclophosphamide
   h. Thiazides
   i. Barbiturates
   j. Narcotics
   k. Tricyclic antidepressants

## CLINICAL MANIFESTATIONS OF HYPOCALCEMIA AND HYPOPARATHYRODISM

1. Tetany (findings generally progress in the following order)
   a. Paresthesias of the lips, fingers, toes, and tongue
   b. Vague muscle cramps
   c. Positive Chvostek's and Trousseau's signs
   d. Carpopedal spasm
   e. Laryngospasm, bronchospasm
   f. Convulsions
2. Dermatologic
   a. Loss of hair
   b. Dry, scaly skin
   c. Eczematous—like dermatitis
   d. Short, brittle nails with ridges
   e. Increased susceptibility for moniliasis
3. Ocular
   a. Lenticular cataracts
   b. Photophobia
   c. Blepharospasm
4. Cardiovascular
   a. Prolonged QT interval
   b. Hypotension
5. Neurologic/Psychiatric
   a. Depression
   b. Anxiety
   c. Emotional lability
   d. Psychosis
   e. Rarely, coma

## CAUSES OF HYPOCALCEMIA

1. Hypoparathyroidism
2. Resistance to parathyroid hormone
   a. Pseudohypoparathyroidism
   b. Magnesium deficiency
3. Disorder of vitamin D metabolism
   a. Diet deficiency
   b. Malabsorption
   c. Drug-induced (anticonvulsants, barbiturates)
   d. Liver disease
   e. Renal disease
4. Malabsorption of calcium and/or vitamin D
5. Removal of calcium from the blood
   a. Osteoblastic metastases (most often, cancer of the prostate)
   b. Acute pancreatitis
   c. Hyperphosphatemia
6. Hypoalbuminemia

# CLINICAL MANIFESTATIONS OF HYPERCALCEMIA AND HYPERPARATHYROIDISM

1. Soft tissue calcification*
   a. Arthropathy
   b. Pseudogout
   c. Conjunctivitis
   d. Corneal calcifications
   e. Pruritis
2. Renal
   a. Nephrocalcinosis
   b. Nephrolithiasis
   c. Polyuria/polydipsia
3. Cardiovascular
   a. ECG changes: shortened QT interval, increased susceptibility to digitalis-toxic arrhythmias, heart block
   b. Hypertension
   c. Cardiac arrest (with hypercalcemic crisis)
4. Gastrointestinal
   a. Anorexia and weight loss
   b. Nausea and vomiting
   c. Constipation
   d. Abdominal discomfort
   e. Peptic ulcer disease
   f. Pancreatitis (acute and chronic)
5. Neurologic
   a. Headache
   b. Lethargy, apathy
   c. Personality changes
   d. Delerium, stupor, coma
6. Muscular and skeletal
   a. Myopathy
   b. Bone pain and tenderness
   c. Spontaneous fractures

*Soft tissue calcification is more often the result of hyperphosphatemia than hypercalcemia, and usually occurs when the Ca × Phosphate product exceeds 40-50 mg/dl².

## CAUSES OF HYPERCALCEMIA

1. Hyperparathyroidism
2. Malignancy
   a. Metastatic destruction of bone (e.g., multiple myeloma, leukemia, lymphoma, breast cancer)
   b. Without bone metastases
      1. Ectopic PTH (most commonly lung and kidney malignancies)
      2. Prostaglandins, osteoclast-activators, other substances
3. Granulomas
   a. Sarcoidosis
   b. Berylliosis
   c. Tuberculosis
   d. Fungal diseases
4. Other, less common, causes
   a. Thyrotoxicosis
   b. Prolonged immobilization (especially patients with Paget's disease)
   c. Vitamin D intoxication
   d. Vitamin A intoxication
   e. Milk-alkali syndrome
   f. Acute renal failure (especially during the recovery phase)
   g. Thiazide diuretics
   h. Addison's disease
   i. Pheochromocytoma
   j. Factitious (prolonged use of tourniquet while drawing blood sample)
   k. Lithium

## USE OF DRUGS IN THE TREATMENT
## OF HYPERCALCEMIA*

Hypercalcemia is managed by:

1. Vigorous hydration to maximize urinary calcium excretion
2. Ambulation or maximizing activity as tolerated
3. Use of drugs to enhance calcium excretion and inhibit bone resorption

| Drug | Onset of effect | Duration of effect | Contraindications (comments) |
|------|-----------------|--------------------|------------------------------|
| Furosemide | 4–8 h | 4–6 h | None |
| Prednisone | 3–6 days | 4–8 days | None, acutely |
| Phosphate IV | 4–8 h | 3–6 days | Renal failure, hyperphosphatemia |
| oral | 2–4 days | 3–6 days | Renal failure, hyperphosphatemia |
| Calcitonin | 6–24 h | 12–24 h | None; effect declines with repeated use |
| Mithramycin | 12–36 h | 1–2 days | Side effects: thrombocytopenia, bleeding disorders, severe marrow toxicity |
| EDTA | ¼–1 h | 1–2 h | Renal failure, frequently causes hypocalcemia |

*Adapted from Clinical Disorders of Fluid and Electrolyte Metabolism, 3rd ed. by Maxwell & Kleeman. Copyright © 1980, McGraw-Hill, New York. Used with the permission of McGraw-Hill Book Company.

## COMMON CAUSES OF SECONDARY HYPERPARATHYROIDISM

1. Chronic renal disease
2. Osteomalacia
   a. Vitamin D deficiency
   b. Malabsorption of vitamin D and calcium
   c. Impaired metabolism of vitamin D
      i. Drug-induced (anticonvulsants, barbiturates)
      ii. Renal disease
      iii. Liver disease
3. Pseudohypoparathyroidism
4. Hypomagnesemia
5. Hyperphosphatemia
6. Fluorosis

## BONE DISEASE: SOME DEFINITIONS

1. *Osteopenia:* decreased density of bone; this is a general descriptive term, and implies no particular pathophysiologic cause or mechanism; thus, for example, both osteomalacia and osteoporosis are forms of osteopenia.
2. *Renal osteodystrophy:* a syndrome of bony changes associated with renal failure and secondary hyperparathyroidism; among the disorders that may be present to varying degrees are osteoporosis, osteomalacia, osteosclerosis, and osteitis fibrosa cystica.
3. *Osteoporosis:* decreased total mass of bone, both mineral and matrix; the ratio of mineral to matrix remains normal; the most common causes include primary disease (postmenopausal or senile), various endocrinopathies (including hyperparathyroidism, hyperthyroidism and Cushing's disease), prolonged immobilization and chronic heparin therapy.
4. *Osteomalacia:* "softening of the bones"; decreased mineral content of bone; most often caused by a deficiency of the active form of vitamin D.
5. *Osteosclerosis:* increased bone density; cause of "rugger jersey spine."
6. *Osteitis fibrosa cystica:* replacement of normal bone by fibrous tissue, usually seen in chronic hemodialysis patients after several years.
7. *Osteogenesis imperfecta:* "brittle bones"; a form of osteoporosis, genetically determined, associated with recurrent fractures and, in the "congenita" form, with blue sclerae.

## FACTORS AFFECTING BONE METABOLISM

1. Matrix synthesis
    a. Increased by
        i. Exertion and exercise
        ii. Chronically increased parathyroid hormone
        iii. Fluoride
    b. Decreased by
        i. Starvation
        ii. Corticosteroids
        iii. Acutely increased parathyroid hormone
        iv. Chronic estrogen deficiency
2. Mineralization
    a. Increased by
        i. High plasma $Ca^{++}$ × phosphate product
        ii. Vitamin D metabolites
    b. Decreased by
        i. Low $Ca^{++}$ × phosphate product
        ii. Vitamin D deficiency
        iii. Diphosphonates
3. Bone resorption
    a. Increased by
        i. Parathyroid hormone
        ii. 1-$\alpha$, 25-Dihydroxycholecalciferol
        iii. 25-Hydroxycholecalciferol
        iv. Thyroxine
        v. Triiodothyronine
        vi. Hypophosphatemia
        vii. Prostaglandin E
        viii. Vitamin A
        ix. Osteoclast activating factor
    b. Decreased by calcitonin
        i. Calcitonin

## CAUSES OF HYPERPHOSPHATEMIA*†

1. Diminished glomerular filtration rate (renal insufficiency)
2. Increased tubular resorption of phosphate
   a. Hypoparathyroidism
   b. Pseudohypothyroidism
   c. Hyperthyroidism
   d. Acromegaly
   e. Diphosphonate therapy of Paget's disease
   f. Tumoral calcinosis
   g. Severe volume contraction
3. Increased phosphate load
   a. Exogenous
      i. Excessive oral phosphate supplementation
      ii. Laxative abuse
      iii. Phosphate enemas
   b. Endogenous
      i. Rhabdomyolysis
      ii. Cell lysis secondary to antineoplastic chemotherapy of leukemia and lymphoma

*Severe hyperphosphatemia (exceeding 10 mg/dl) is almost always due to an increased phosphate load.
†The predominant signs and symptoms of hyperphosphatemia are those of hypocalcemia, secondary hyperparathyroidism, and metastatic soft tissue calcification.

## CAUSES OF HYPOPHOSPHATEMIA

### I. Notes

1. The most common settings for hypophosphatemia are
   a. Alcoholism
   b. Decompensated diabetes mellitus
   c. Hyperalimentation with inadequate phosphate replenishment
   d. Refeeding after prolonged starvation
   e. Respiratory alkalosis
2. Malabsorption causes hypophosphatemia predominantly on the basis of secondary hyperparathyroidism (due to calcium and vitamin D deficiency) and not inadequate absorption of phosphate
3. The major consequences of hypophosphatemia are:
   a. Decreased red cell, white cell, and platelet function
   b. Osteomalacia
   c. Myopathy
   d. Metabolic encephalopathy

### II. Etiologies

1. Inadequate intake
   a. Starvation
   b. Excessive use of aluminum-containing antacids
2. Excessive renal losses
   a. Primary and secondary hyperparathyroidism
   b. Glycosuria
   c. Vitamin D deficiency
   d. Fanconi's syndrome
   e. Malabsorption
   f. Volume expansion
   g. Hypomagnesemia
   h. Diuretics
3. Excessive GI losses
   a. Chronic diarrhea
   b. Severe vomiting
4. Transport of phosphate into cells
   a. Glucose administration
   b. Insulin administration
   c. Respiratory alkalosis

5. Alcoholism
   a. Upon admission (due to inadequate intake, diarrhea, vomiting, hypomagnesemia, and secondary hyperparathyroidism; secondary hyperparathyroidism in alcoholics is generally due to calcium and vitamin D deficiency)
   b. Twelve to 48 hours after admission (due to glucose refeeding and the onset of respiratory alkalosis with withdrawal)

## CAUSES OF HYPOGLYCEMIA
## IN THE DIABETIC PATIENT
### (In Order of Decreasing Frequency)

1. Insufficient carbohydrate intake (by far the most common cause of hypoglycemia in these patients)
2. Excessive dose of insulin or a sulfonylurea (accidental or intentional)
3. Strenuous exercise or other stress (infection, surgery, emotional trauma)
4. Excessive alcohol intake
5. Less common causes
   a. Failure to adjust insulin or sulfonylurea dosage despite worsening renal failure
   b. Failure to adjust insulin dosage despite worsening liver failure
   c. Reduction in corticosteroid dosage
   d. Drugs that increase insulin release
      i. $\alpha$-Antagonists
      ii. $\beta$-Agonists
      iii. MAO-Inhibitors
   e. Drugs that potentiate the action of sulfonylureas

   | | |
   |---|---|
   | i. Salicylates | vi. Barbiturates |
   | ii. Sulfonamides | vii. Probenecid |
   | iii. Propranolol | viii. Chloramphenicol |
   | iv. Clofibrate | ix. MAO inhibitors |
   | v. Phenylbutazone | x. Bishydroxy coumarin |

## CAUSES OF HYPOGLYCEMIA IN THE NONDIABETIC PATIENT

1. Fasting hypoglycemia
   a. Alcoholism
   b. Liver disease
   c. Uremia
   d. Congestive heart failure
   e. Hormonal
      i. Adrenal insufficiency
      ii. Deficiency of glucagon, epinephrine, or growth hormone
   f. Malnutrition
   g. Insulinoma
   h. Nonpancreatic tumors
      i. Sarcomas of the retroperitoneum, abdomen, and thorax
      ii. Hepatomas
      iii. Widely metastatic cancer
   i. Strenuous exercise
2. Postprandial hypoglycemia
   a. Reactive hypoglycemia
   b. Alimentary hypoglycemia (dumping syndrome)
   c. Latent diabetes mellitus
   d. Hormonal (as above)
3. Factitious hypoglycemia

## THE STAGES OF HYPOGLYCEMIA:
## SIGNS AND SYMPTOMS

1. Adrenergic stage: palpitations, diaphoresis, hyperventilation, anxiety, faintness, tremulousness, weakness, hunger, nausea
2. Cortical stage
   a. Headache, confusion, altered behavior, hallucinations
   b. Abnormal reflexes, primitive movements, transient paralysis, hypothermia, convulsions
3. Medullary stage: bradycardia, shallow and slowed respirations, meiosis, pupils unreactive to light, pallor, hyporeflexia, flaccidity, coma

## COMMON INSULIN PREPARATIONS

| Preparation | Type of Suspension | Onset of Activity* | Peak Activity* | Duration of Activity* |
|---|---|---|---|---|
| *Rapid-acting* | | | | |
| Regular | Solution | ¼–½ | 4-6 | 6-8 |
| Semilente | Amorphous | ½–1 | 4-6 | 12-16 |
| *Intermediate-acting* | | | | |
| Globin | Solution | 2-3 | 6-10 | 12-18 |
| NPH | Crystalline | 3 | 8-12 | 18-24 |
| Lente | 30% amorphous, 70% crystalline | 3 | 8-12 | 18-24 |
| *Slow-acting* | | | | |
| Protamine zinc (PZI) | Amorphous | 3 | 14-20 | 24-36 |
| Ultralente | Crystalline | 3-4 | 16-18 | 30-36 |

*Hours after subcutaneous injection.

## THE METABOLIC EFFECTS OF INSULIN AND INSULIN DEFICIENCY

| Tissue | High insulin (fed) state | Low insulin (fasting) state | Insulin deficiency (diabetes) |
|---|---|---|---|
| Adipose | Insulin inhibits lipolysis, promotes lipid synthesis and storage, as well as free fatty acid and glucose uptake | Glucose and lipid uptake are decreased; lipid is degraded into free fatty acids which are released into the circulation | Excessive release of free fatty acids and inhibition of glucose uptake |
| Muscle | Insulin promotes glucose and amino acid uptake, as well as protein and glycogen synthesis | Glucose uptake is decreased, and amino acids are released into the circulation | Excessive release of amino acids and inhibition of glucose uptake |
| Liver | Insulin promotes glucose uptake and glycogen synthesis while shutting off gluconeogenesis; also promotes lipogenesis and inhibits ketogenesis | Glycogenolysis and gluconeogenesis keep blood glucose levels elevated; sufficient insulin is present to prevent excessive ketogenesis | Excessive gluconeogenesis plus failure of glucose uptake by insulin-sensitive tissues leads to hyperglycemia. In DKA (but not in hyperosmolar coma) free fatty acids are oxidized to ketone bodies beyond the body's ability to consume them |

## CHRONIC COMPLICATIONS OF DIABETES MELLITUS

1. Infection
2. Renal disease
   a. Glomerulosclerosis (the Kimmelstiel-Wilson lesion is a nodular glomerulosclerosis)
   b. Papillary necrosis
   c. Pyelonephritis
   d. Hypertension
   e. Renal artery arteriosclerosis
   f. Increased risk of acute failure following angiographic procedures.
3. Eye disease
   a. Retinopathy (nonproliferative and proliferative)
   b. Glaucoma
   c. Cataracts
4. Cardiovascular disease
   a. Peripheral atherosclerosis (both large and small vessels)
      i. Claudication
      ii. Ulceration
      iii. Infection (amputation for gangrene accounts for nearly half of all operations among diabetics)
   b. Coronary atherosclerosis (infarctions may be silent)
   c. Diabetic cardiomyopathy
5. Neurologic disease
   a. Peripheral neuropathy (the most common neurologic lesion among diabetics is bilateral symmetric sensory impairment, usually of the lower extremities, consisting of anesthesia and diminshed reflexes, although hyperesthesia and burning pain may also occur, typically at night)
   b. Mononeuropathy simplex or multiplex (transient lesions affecting the extraocular muscles are most common)

## CHRONIC COMPLICATIONS OF
## DIABETES MELLITUS *(cont.)*

c. Automatic neuropathy
   i. Cardiovascular: tachycardia, loss of normal sinus arrhythmia, orthostatic hypotension, syncope
   ii. Gastrointestinal: gastric dilation and impaired GI motility (gastroparesis), hyperemesis, diarrhea, constipation
   iii. Neurogenic bladder
   iv. Sexual impotence
   v. Loss of sweating
d. Diabetic amyotrophy (pelvic muscle tenderness, waddling gait)
e. Charcot joints
f. Neuropathic ulcers

## COMMON ERRORS IN MANAGING DIABETIC KETOACIDOSIS*

1. Insufficient replacement of fluids and electrolytes (fluid overload in elderly diabetics, however, is hazardous)
2. Inadequate insulin at infrequent intervals
3. Unnecessary or excessive use of bicarbonate
4. Excessive dosage of IV insulin (receptors are fully saturated with 7–10 units)
5. Failure to replete potassium losses adequately
6. Failure to begin D5W when the blood glucose drops to 250–300 mg/100 ml
7. Failure to recognize delayed hypoglycemia
8. Premature cessation of insulin therapy
9. Failure to give diet and intermediate-acting insulins after ketosis has cleared

*Adapted from MGH Textbook of Emergency Medicine, ed. Earle W. Wilkins, Jr. p. 232. © 1978, the Williams & Wilkins Co., Baltimore.

## DIABETIC COMA: HYPOGLYCEMIA
## VS. KETOACIDOSIS

|  | *Hypoglycemia* | *Ketoacidosis* |
|---|---|---|
| *Common Precipitants* | Diminished food intake | Infection |
|  | Excessive use of insulin or a sulfonylurea | Diminished use of insulin or a sulfonylurea |
|  | Strenuous exercise | Myocardial infarction |
|  | Excessive alcohol intake | Pregnancy |
|  | Stress of any kind | Abdominal catastrophe |
|  | Renal failure without reduction of insulin dosage |  |

### *Preceding history*

|  | | |
|---|---|---|
| Onset of coma | Minutes | Hours to days |
| Nausea, vomiting, abdominal pain | Uncommon | Common |
| Polyuria, polydipsia | No | Yes |
| Tremulousness | Yes | No |
| Altered behavior | Yes | No |

### *Physical examination*

|  | | |
|---|---|---|
| Temperature | Normal or decreased | Normal or decreased |
| Pulse | Rapid | Rapid |
| Blood pressure | Normal or increased | Decreased |
| Respirations | Shallow | Deep and rapid |
| Sweating | Increased | Decreased |
| Hydration | Normal | Decreased |
| CNS signs | Any pattern may be seen | Generalized depressed function |

### *Laboratory*

|  | | |
|---|---|---|
| Urine glucose | − or + (not helpful) | + |
| Urine acetone | − or + (not helpful) | + |
| Blood glucose | Normal or low | Increased |
| Blood acetone | − | + |
| Arterial pH | Normal | Acidosis |
| Plasma bicarbonate | Normal | Decreased |

## IMPORTANT CAUSES OF GYNECOMASTIA

1. Normal puberty
2. Senescence
3. Obesity
4. Neoplasms
   a. Gonadotropin-secreting (lung, adrenal, testes, liver)
   b. Estrogen-secreting (adrenal, testes)
   c. Pituitary tumors
   d. Hodgkin's disease
5. Endocrine disorders
   a. Hyperthyroidism
   b. Hypothyroidism
   c. Cushing's syndrome
   d. Testicular failure
   e. Klinefelter's syndrome
   f. Reifenstein's syndrome
6. Refeeding after severe malnutrition, starvation, or chronic illness
7. Chronic hemodialysis for renal failure
8. Severe liver disease (especially alcoholic cirrhosis)
9. Ulcerative colitis
10. Drugs
    a. Estrogens
    b. Gonadotropins
    c. Marijuana
    d. Digitalis
    e. Isoniazid
    f. Phenothiazines
    g. Reserpine
    h. Spironolactone
    i. Meprobamate
    j. Cimetidine

## THYROID FUNCTION TESTS

1. Total serum thyroxine (T4)
   a. Method: radioimmunoasssay or competitive protein binding
   b. Normal value: 5–12 ug/dl
   c. Interpretation: This is the standard screen for thyroid disease, successfully diagnosing 90% of all cases of hyperthyroidism and 85% of all cases of hypothyroidism. However, the value varies with fluctuating levels of thyroid-binding proteins. Thus, an elevated total serum T4 may be due solely to an increase in the concentration of thyroxine-binding globulin (TBG), although the concentration of unbound (active) hormone is normal and the patient is euthyroid.

### Causes of Variations in TBG Concentration

| *Increased* | *Decreased* |
| --- | --- |
| Estrogens, oral contraceptives | Androgens, glucocorticoids |
| Pregnancy | Nephrotic syndrome |
| Heroin | Hypoproteinemia (e.g. protein-losing enteropathy) |
| Liver disease | Severe illness |
| Genetic tendency | Liver disease |
| | Acromegaly |
| | Cushing's syndrome |
| | Genetic tendency |

2. Total serum T3
   a. Method: radioimmunoassay
   b. Normal value: 80–160 ng/dl
   c. Interpretation: The serum T3 usually varies in concert with the serum T4, but there are some situations in which this need not be true:
      i. The T3 alone may be elevated early in hyperthyroidism and in the syndrome of "T3 toxicosis."
      ii. Approximately half of all hypothyroid patients have a normal serum T3.
      iii. The T3 can be decreased in euthyroid patients suffering from severe illnesses, especially malnutrition, uremia cirrhosis.
3. T3 resin uptake (RT3U)
   a. Method: The patient's serum is incubated with radiolabelled T3 solid resin. The amount of label bound to the resin is inversely proportional to the binding sites available in the patient's serum

b. Normal value: 25–35% of the total radioactivity is ground to the resin

Interpretation: Used to distinguish thyroid disorders from alterations in thyroid binding proteins. A low uptake is compatible with low hormone levels or an increased number of binding sites available (increased TBG). A high uptake is compatible with elevated hormone levels or a decreased number of available binding sites (decreased TBG). A *free T4 index* can be calculated by multiplying the RT3U by the total T4 (similarly, RT3U × T3 gives the free T3 index). This value is an excellent approximation of the concentration of free hormone in the patient's serum.

*(The normal free T4 index is 1.5–3.6)*

| Total T4 | RT3U | Free T4 index | Cause |
|---|---|---|---|
| Incr. | Incr. | Incr. | Hyperthyroidism |
| Decr. | Decr. | Decr. | Hypothyroidism |
| Incr. | Decr. | Approx. nl | Increased TBG |
| Decr. | Incr. | Approx. nl | Decreased TBG |

4. Free T4

Method: equilibrium dialysis

Normal value:1–4 ng/dl

Interpretation: This test gives a direct measurement of active thyroxine, independent of TBG concentrations.

5. TSH testing

Method: radioimmunoassay

Normal value: 0–6 $\mu$g/ml

Interpretation: This is the most sensitive test for hypothyroidism. TSH levels are virtually always elevated in primary hypothyroidism.

6. TRH stimulation test

Method: measures release of TSH in response to IV TRH

Normal value: at least a twofold increase in TSH

Interpretation: When hypothyroidism is suspected on clinical grounds in a patient with low levels of TSH, this test can be used to assess a possible hypothalamic or pituitary origin.

7. Thyroid scan

Method: scan with $^{123}$I or $^{99m}$Tc

Interpretation: Best diagnostic tool for studying thyroid nodules. "Hot" (functioning) nodules are rarely malignant.

8. Other tests

a. Ultrasonography: excellent for distinguishing solid from cystic nodules; the latter are rarely malignant

## THYROID FUNCTION TESTS *(cont.)*

    b. Anti-thyroid antibodies: when present in high titers, these suggest Hashimoto's thyroiditis

    c. TSIg can be used to distinguish Graves' disease from other forms of hyperthyroidism

Special notes

    a. Phenytoin decreases both total and free T4 measurements, although the patient is euthyroid; heparin increases these values.

    b. Patients with chronic renal failure frequently have a decreased T3, normal T4, and a normal or mildly elevated TSH.

## DIAGNOSTIC STRATEGIES

## Strategy for Evaluation of Possible Hyperthyroidism

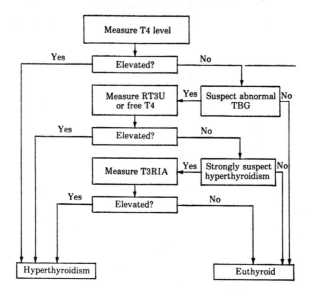

## Strategy for Evaluation of Possible Hypothyroidism

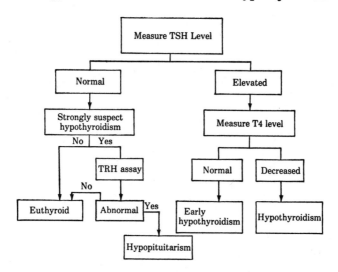

## DIAGNOSTIC STRATEGIES *(cont.)*

### Strategy for Evaluation of Clinically Euthyroid Patient with Thyroid Nodule

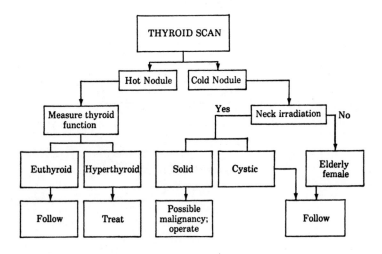

## CLINICAL MANIFESTATIONS OF HYPOTHYROIDISM

1. Very common (present in more than 80% of patients)
   a. Dry, coarse, cold skin
   b. Cold intolerance
   c. Lethargy, tiredness
   d. Slow speech
   e. Periorbital edema
   f. Decreased sweating
2. Usually present (>50%)
   a. Coarse, brittle hair with patchy alopecia
   b. Puffiness of face, hands, feet
   c. Thick tongue
   d. Hoarseness
   e. Weight gain
   f. Constipation
   g. Impaired memory
   h. Delay in relaxation phase of deep tendon reflexes
   i. Goiter
   j. Loss of outer third of eyebrows
3. Less common (<50%)
   a. Arthralgias and myalgias
   b. Bradycardia
   c. Hypertension
   d. Palpitations
   e. Chest pain
   f. Paresthesias
   g. Myxedema "madness" and myxedema "wit"
   h. Menorrhagia or amenorrhea
   i. Anorexia
   j. Deafness
   k. Fluid accumulations (pleural, pericardial, ascites)

## CAUSES OF HYPOTHYROIDISM

1. Iatrogenic
   a. Postthyroidectomy
   b. Radioactive iodine therapy for thyrotoxicosis
   c. Irradiation for tumors of head, neck, upper thorax
   d. SSKI and other iodine-containing agents
   e. Lithium therapy for manic-depressive disorders
2. Hashimoto's thyroiditis
3. Hypothyroidism of Graves' disease and subacute thyroiditis
4. Iodine deficiency
5. Iodine excess
6. Infiltrative disease (e.g., sarcoidosis)
7. Deficiency of TRH (hypothalmic disease)
8. Deficiency of TSH (hypopituitarism)
9. Biosynthetic defects in thyroid hormonogenesis
10. Peripheral resistance to thyroid hormone

## CLINICAL MANIFESTATIONS
## OF HYPERTHYROIDISM*

1. Very common (present in more than 80% of patients)
   a. Warm, moist skin
   b. Heat intolerance
   c. Nervousness, hyperkinesia
   d. Fine tremor (best seen with outstretched hands)
   e. Bruit over the thyroid gland
   f. Weight loss
   g. Palpitations, tachycardia, systolic flow murmur
   h. Fatigue
   i. Goiter
2. Usually present (>50%)
   a. Ocular findings: lid lag, stare, and exophthalmos (the last confined to Graves' disease) cause burning, tearing, diplopia, and diminished visual acuity
   b. Polyphagia
   c. Dyspnea
   d. Proximal muscle weakness
   e. Hyperactive reflexes
3. Less common (<50%)
   a. Chest pain
   b. Gynecomastia
   c. Arrhythmias (especially atrial fibrillation)
   d. Swelling of legs
   e. Increased frequency of bowel movements with or without diarrhea
   f. Splenomegaly
   g. Vitiligo
   h. Liver palms
   i. Pruritis
   j. Loss of hair
   k. Pretibial myxedema (only in Graves' disease)

*Elderly patients may present with "apathetic thyrotoxicosis," marked by depression, cachexia, anorexia, and constipation. The only clues to the presence of hyperthyroidism may be moderate tachycardia and weakness, new onset arrhythmias, or otherwise unexplained worsening of angina or CHF.

## CAUSES OF HYPERTHYROIDISM

1. Graves' disease
2. Subacute thyroiditis
3. Toxic multinodular goiter
4. Single follicular adenomas
5. Jod-Basedow's phenomenon (iodine-induced thyrotoxicosis in a patient with preexisting goiter)
6. Toxic thyroid carcinoma
7. Pituitary tumors (producing TSH)
8. Struma ovarii
9. Hydatidiform moles (producing HCG)
10. Thyrotoxicosis factitia (due to excess exogenous hormone)

## THYROID CARCINOMA

1. Papillary carcinoma
   a. Pathology: fronds of cells containing little colloid; the majority of tumors contain some normal follicular strucutres
   b. Prevalence: 50–75% of all thyroid carcinomas
   c. Average age of onset: bimodal, with peaks at 10–30 and in the elderly
   d. Sex ratio: 3 females : 1 male
   e. Metastases: slow growing; early metastases via lymphatics to the gland itself and local nodes where it remains indolent for many years; later may spread to larynx, lungs
   f. Ten year survival: 80–90%
2. Follicular carcinoma
   a. Pathology: may appear like normal thyroid or contain follicles of varying sizes
   b. Prevalence: 15–20%
   c. Average age of onset: 50 years
   d. Sex ratio: 2–3 female : 1 male
   e. Metastases: more aggressive than papillary tumors; metastasizes early via the blood to the lung, bones, rarely to the local nodes; later may spread to the CNS
   f. Ten-year survival: 50%
   g. Comment: actively takes up iodine, may suppress; may rarely cause thyrotoxicosis
3. Anaplastic tumors
   a. Pathology: varied, undifferentiated
   b. Prevalence: 10%
   c. Average age of onset: greater than 60 years
   d. Sex ratio: equal
   e. Metastases: very aggressive; invades locally (causing pain, hemoptysis, hoarseness, dysphagia) and spreads widely
   f. Ten-year survival: rare—death usually occurs within one year
4. Medullary carcinoma
   a. Pathology: sheets of "C" cells
   b. Prevalence: 1–5%
   c. Average age of onset: 50 years
   d. Sex ratio: slightly more common in females
   e. Metastases: local spread to neck, then to soft tissues, lungs
   f. Ten-year survival: 90%
   g. Comment: associated with multiple endocrine syndromes (MEN II); secretes calcitonin, but rarely causes hypocalcemia; some secrete ACTH and can cause Cushing's syndrome

## CLINICAL MANIFESTATIONS OF
## ADDISON'S DISEASE

1. Common (present in the majority of patients)
   a. Weakness, fatigue, lethargy
   b. Hyperpigmentation*
   c. Hyponatremia*
   d. Hyperkalemia*
   e. Orthostatic hypotension
   f. Dehydration
   g. Nausea, vomiting, anorexia, weight loss
   h. Elevated eosinophil count
2. Less common
   a. Myalgias, arthralgias
   b. Vitiligo*
   c. Abdominal pain
   d. Diarrhea
   e. Loss of body hair
   f. Sexual dysfunction, amenorrhea
   g. Depression, psychosis
   h. Salt craving*
   i. Hypoglycemia
3. Laboratory confirmation
   a. Decreased 24-hour urinary free cortisol and 17-hydroxycorticosteroids
   b. Decreased cortisol response to ACTH stimulation (only to primary disease)

*Seen only in primary (adrenal) Addison's disease.

## CAUSES OF ADDISON'S DISEASE

1. Primary (adrenal) disease
   a. Autoimmune
   b. Idiopathic
   c. Infection (especially tuberculosis)
   d. Hemorrhage (sepsis, trauma, anticoagulant therapy)
   e. Infiltrative disease (tumors, leukemia, amyloidosis)
2. Hypopituitarism
3. Hypothalamic disease

The most common setting for Addisonian crisis is the patient on chronic steroid therapy. Suppression of the hypothalamic-pituitary-adrenal axis leads to adrenal atrophy, and the adrenal gland is unable to produce and release hormone when confronted with stress. Probably the second leading cause is an acute bleed into the adrenal gland. Patients in Addisonian crisis present with shock and severe back pain.

## CAUSES OF CUSHING'S SYNDROME

1. Adrenal tumors
   a. Adenomas
   b. Carcinomas
2. Cushing's disease (bilateral adrenal hyperplasia due to a pituitary adenoma secreting ACTH)
3. Ectopic ACTH production
   a. Lung cancer (especially oat cell carcinoma)
   b. Thymic tumors
   c. Pancreatic islet cell tumors
   d. Renal cell tumors
4. Chronic steroid therapy
5. Pseudo-Cushing's syndrome (seen in alcoholics)

## CUSHING'S SYNDROME:
## HELPFUL LABORATORY FINDINGS

| | Serum ACTH levels | Low dose dexamethasone | High dose dexamethasone |
|---|---|---|---|
| Adrenal tumors | Low | No suppression | No suppression |
| Cushing's disease | High | No suppression | Suppression |
| Ectopic ACTH | High | No suppression | No suppression |

In patients with primary adrenal Cushing's syndrome, it is usually possible to distinguish adenomas from carcinomas on the basis of androgen production. With a few reported exceptions, only carcinomas produce androgens and will have elevated urinary 17-ketosteroids. Adenomas are much more common.

## CLINICAL MANIFESTATIONS OF CUSHING'S SYNDROME

1. Common (present in the majority of patients)
   a. Central obesity (with a "buffalo hump" and supraclavicular fat pad)
   b. Moon facies
   c. Striae
   d. Easy bruisability
   e. Hypertension
   f. Menstrual or sexual dysfunction
   g. Virilization (hirsutism, acne, deep voice, balding)
   h. Osteoporosis
   i. Mental changes (depression, euphoria)
   k. Impaired glucose tolerance
2. Less common
   a. Muscle weakness or atrophy
   b. Edema of lower extremities
   c. Aseptic necrosis of bone
   d. Vertebral fractures
   e. Kidney stones
   f. Diabetes mellitus
   g. Fungal infections of the skin
   h. Cataracts or glaucoma
   i. Psychosis
   j. Hypokalemia
3. Laboratory Studies
   a. Best screen: overnight dexamethasone suppression test
   b. Confirm
      i. Elevated urinary free cortisol and 17-hydroxycorticosteroids
      ii. Loss of normal diurnal variation of serum costisol levels

# HYPERLIPIDEMIAS

1. Are lipid levels elevated?

|  | *Cholesterol* | *Triglycerides* |
|---|---|---|
| 45-year-old male | >270 mg/100 ml | >160 mg/100 ml |
| 45-year-old female | >240 mg/100 ml | >140 mg/100 ml |

2. Is plasma cloudy? After cooling, examine.
   a. A creamy ring of fat on top indicates elevated chylomicrons.
   b. Cloudy plasma indicates elevated VLDL.
   c. Clear plasma without refractile material indicates elevated LDL.
3. What is the primary disorder? Electrophoretic pattern helps define epidemiology, likely sequelae.

## Classification

| Disorder | Electro-phoretic pattern | Frequency | Abnormality | |
|---|---|---|---|---|
|  |  |  | LIPID | LIPO-PROTEIN |
| Familial lipo-protein lipase deficiency | I | Very rare | TG* | CM† |
| Familial hyper-cholesterolemia | IIa IIb | 0.1–0.5% | Chol‡ TG Chol | LDL LDL VLDL |
| Polygenic hyper-cholesterolemia | II | 5% | Chol | LDL |
| Familial dys-betalipopro-teinemia | III | Rare | TG, Chol | Broad band β-lipopro-protein |
| Familial hyper-triglyderidemia | IV | 1–2% (most common) | TG | VLDL |
|  | V | Uncommon | TG | CM, VLDL |
| Familial com-bined hyper-lipidemia | IIa, IIb, IV | 1–2% | TG, Chol | Abnormal glucose tolerance |

*TG = triglyceride
†CM = chylomicrons
‡Chol = cholesterol

## HYPERLIPIDEMIAS *(cont.)*

| Familial hyper-triglyceridemia | Cloudy | High | Tuberous xanthomas, pancreatitis, abnormal glucose tolerance |
|---|---|---|---|
| (Type V) | Cloudy with creamy layer on top | Possibly high | Eruptive xanthomas, pancreatitis, hepato-splenomegaly, ab-dominal pain, abnor-mal glucose tolerance |
| Familial com-bined hyper-lipidemia | IIa, IIb, IV | 1–2% | TG, Chol |

### Clinical Recognition and Significance

| Disorder | Plasma Appearance | Risk of ASCVD | Clinical Manifestations |
|---|---|---|---|
| Familial lipo-protein lipase deficiency | Creamy layer on top, clear below | Low | Eruptive xanthomas, pancreatitis, hepato-splenomegaly, ab-dominal pain |
| Familial hyper-cholestero-lemia | (IIA) clear (IIB) cloudy | Very high | Tuberous and tendon-ous xanthomas, xanthelasma, cor-neal arcus |
| Polygenic hy-percholester-olemia | Clear | High | Tuberous and tendon-ous xanthomas, xanthelasma, cor-neal arcus |
| Familial dys-betalipopro-teinemia | Cloudy, +/− creamy layer | Very high | Palmar, tuberous, or tendonous xanthomas |

## HYPERLIPIDEMIAS *(cont.)*

**Secondary Hyperlipidemic States: Alteration in Serum Cholesterol and Triglycerides due to Underlying Diseases**

|  | *Cholesterol* | *Triglycerides* |
|---|---|---|
| Hypothyroidism | Increased | Increased or normal |
| Nephrotic syndrome | Increased | Increased or normal |
| Biliary cirrhosis | Increased | Increased or normal |
| Diabetes mellitus | Normal | Increased |
| Alcoholism | Normal | Increased |
| Uremia | Normal | Increased |
| Birth control pills | Normal | Increased |
| Pregnancy | Normal | Increased |
| Dysgammaglobulinemia | Increased or nl | Increased or normal |
| Obesity | Normal | Increased |
| Hyperuricemia | Normal | Increased |
| Hypertension | Normal | Increased |

## VITAMINS

1. Vitamin A
   a. Synonym: retinol
   b. Solubility: fat-soluble
   c. Best sources: liver, vegetables, dairy products
   d. Deficiency
      i. Eye and skin lesions (especially night blindness, xerophthalmia, hyperkeratosis and keratomalacia)
      ii. Diminished resistance to infection
   e. Toxicity
      i. Acute: drowsiness, irritability, headache, nausea and vomiting.
      ii. Chronic: bone and joint pain, hair loss, hepatomegaly, anorexia and weight loss, increased CSF pressure, dryness, and cracking of lips
   f. Recommended daily adult allowance: 5,000 IU
2. Vitamin $B_1$
   a. Synonym: thiamine
   b. Solubility: water-soluble
   c. Best sources: whole grains, meats, leafy vegetables, legumes
   d. Deficiency: beriberi
      i. Cardiovascular manifestations: high-output failure
      ii. Neurologic manifestations: peripheral neuropathy, Wernicke's encephalopathy, Korsakoff syndrome
   e. Toxicity: edema, nervousness, tremors, sweating, tachycardia, hypotension
   f. Recommended daily adult allowance: 1.0–1.4 mg
3. Vitamin $B_2$
   a. Synonym: riboflavin
   b. Solubility: water-soluble
   c. Best sources: organ meats, leafy vegetables, meats, fish, eggs, milk, nuts
   d. Deficiency: mucosal lesions, especially of the lips, mouth, and tongue, and seborrheic dermatitis
   e. Toxicity: none
   f. Recommended daily adult allowance: 2.0 mg
4. Vitamin $B_6$
   a. Synonym: pyridoxine
   b. Solubility: water-soluble
   c. Best sources: liver, herring, salmon, nuts, brown rice, wheat germ, eggs, butter, many vegetables, meat, fish, some fruits (bananas, grapes, pears)

    d. Deficiency: anemia, skin lesions, seizures and peripheral neuritis

    e. Toxicity: seizures

    f. Recommended daily adult allowance: 2.0–2.5 mg

5. Vitamin $B_{12}$
   a. Synonym: cyanocobalamin
   b. Solubility: water-soluble
   c. Best sources: organ meats, eggs, fish*
   d. Deficiency: megaloblastic anemia, glossitis, subacute combined degeneration (disease of the lateral and dorsal spinal columns), and amenorrhea
   e. Toxicity: reports of polycythemia
   f. Recommended daily adult allowance: 3.0 $\mu$g

6. Folic acid
   a. Synonym: pteroylmonoglutamic acid
   b. Solubility: water-soluble
   c. Best sources: liver, asparagus, spinach, wheat, bran, dry beans, many other vegetables, nuts, grains
   d. Deficiency: megaloblastic anemia
   e. Toxicity: none
   f. Recommended daily adult allowance: 400 $\mu$g

7. Vitamin C
   a. Synonym: ascorbic acid
   b. Solubility: water-soluble
   c. Best sources: citrus fruits, strawberries, many vegetables
   d. Deficiency: scurvy
      i. Malaise and weakness
      ii. Hemorrhages (perifollicular hemorrhages, petechiae, ecchymoses, hemarthroses)
      iii. Gum disease
      iv. Diminished resistance to infection
   e. Toxicity: hyperuricemia and kidney stones
   f. Recommended daily adult allowance: 50–75 mg

8. Vitamin D
   a. Synonym: ergocalciferol or cholecalciferol
   b. Solubility: fat-soluble
   c. Best sources: sunlight, liver oils, eggs, many fish, margarine, dairy products
   d. Deficiency
      i. In adults—osteomalacia
      ii. In children—rickets
   e. Toxicity: hypercalcemia with ectopic calcification
   f. Recommended daily adult allowance: 400 IU

*Only foods of animal origin.

---
## VITAMINS *(cont.)*
---

9. Vitamin E
   a. Synonym: $\alpha$, $\beta$ and $\gamma$ tocopherols
   b. Solubility: fat-soluble
   c. Best sources: oils, margarine, grains, peanuts, many vegetables (especially cabbage, spinach, asparagus)
   d. Deficiency: diminished resistance of red blood cells to oxidative stress
   e. Toxicity: none
   f. Recommended daily adult allowance: 10–15 mg
10. Vitamin K
   a. Synonym: none
   b. Solubility: fat-soluble
   c. Best sources: green leafy vegetables, meats, dairy products
   d. Deficiency: coagulopathy (depletion of clothing factors II, VII, IX, and X)
   e. Toxicity: red blood cell hemolysis with oxidative stress
   f. Recommended daily adult allowance: 70–140 $\mu$g
11. Niacin
   a. Synonym: nicotinic acid
   b. Solubility: water-soluble
   c. Best sources: organ meats, peanuts, rice bran, fish, meats, nuts, vegetables, whole grains
   d. Deficiency: pellagra
      i. Photosensitive dermatitis
      ii. Dementia
      iii. Diarrhea
      iv. Mucosal lesions (including glossitis, stomatitis, achlorhydria, and vaginitis)
   e. Toxicity: peripheral vasodilatation, pruritis and skin rash, nausea, vomiting, diarrhea, heartburn
   f. Recommended daily adult allowance: 15–20 mg
12. Pantothenic acid
   a. Synonym: calcium pantothenate or alcohol panthenol
   b. Solubility: water-soluble
   c. Best sources: organ meats, eggs, herring, wheat germ, bran, peanuts, many vegetables, meats, walnuts, fish
   d. Deficiency: diminished antibody formation (increased susceptibility to infection), and neuropathy
   e. Toxicity: none
   f. Recommended daily adult allowance: 5–10 mg

# Section

# 4

# Hematology

## TRANSFUSIONS: WHOLE BLOOD VS. PACKED CELLS

| | Whole blood | Packed Cells |
|---|---|---|
| Most common clinical use | Acute blood loss, volume replacement | Anemia; used in combination with crystalloid in acute blood loss for volume replacement |

### Composition/Unit

| | Whole blood | Packed Cells |
|---|---|---|
| Volume | 517.5 mL | 300 mL |
| RBC mass | 200 mL | 200 mL |
| Hemoglobin | 30 gm | 30 gm |
| Hematocrit | 40% | 70% |
| Plasma | 250 mL | 78 mL |
| Citrate | 65 | ~22 mL |
| $Na^+$ | 45 mEq | 15 mEq |
| $K^+$ | 15 mEq | 4 mEq |
| Total protein | 48 gm | 36 gm |
| Albumin | 12 gm | 4 gm |

| | | WASHED | FROZEN |
|---|---|---|---|
| *Incidence of hepatitis transmission* | 0.2–0.7% | <0.1% | 0% |
| *Advantages* | Least expensive | Removes allergens | Can store rare blood types for years |
| *Disadvantages* | High incidence of allergic and febrile reactions; increased incidence of hepatitis | Washing introduces potential source of bacterial contamination | Most expensive |
| *Ability to replace* | | | |
| Granulocytes | Lost by 24 hours | Like whole blood | Poor |
| Platelets | Lost by 72 hours | Like whole blood | Poor |
| Coagulation factors | Factors V and VIII lost by 7 days | Like whole blood | Excellent, except low in fibrinogen |

## TRANSFUSION REACTIONS AND COMPLICATIONS

1. Febrile reactions
   a. Incidence: most common transfusion reaction (approximately 2% of transfusions)
   b. Etiology: Presence of leukoagglutinins or platelet agglutinins
   c. Symptoms: usually mild, can include chills, fever, malaise, headache; symptoms usually require transfusion of more than half a unit
   d. Therapy:
      i. Transfusion does not have to be stopped
      ii. Check crossmatch—symptoms may be those of early hemolytic reaction
      iii. Give antipyretics, observe closely
2. Reaction to bacterial contamination
   a. Incidence: rare
   b. Symptoms: severe, can include pain, vomiting, delirium, hypotension, shock; mortality exceeds 50%
   c. Therapy
      i. Stop transfusion
      ii. Draw blood cultures
      iii. Severe reaction necessitates broad antibiotic coverage before culture results are learned
3. Acute hemolysis
   a. Incidence: uncommon with careful crossmatching
   b. Etiology: immunologic incompatibility between donor and recipient blood
   c. Symptoms: early symptoms are indistinguishable from a febrile reaction, but may occur earlier in the transfusion; later symptoms may include nausea, vomiting, hypotension, back and flank pain, and bleeding from IV sites; renal failure, shock, and DIC may eventually develop
   d. Therapy
      i. Check crossmatch, examine plasma and urine for free hemoglobin (both appear red)
      ii. If hemolysis is suspected, stop transfusion, repeat type and crossmatch, obtain hematocrit, haptoglobin, PT, PTT, platelet count, and fibrinogen and fibrin split products
      iii. Support blood pressure, monitor urine output
      iv. Some clinicians give a bolus of 20% mannitol to maintain renal blood flow

4. Allergic (immediate hypersensitivity) reactions
   a. Incidence: common (approximately 4% of transfusions), especially in patients who are IgA deficient
   b. Etiology: reaction to allergens present in donor blood
   c. Symptoms: usually mild, can include fever, bronchospasm, urticaria, pruritis, and angioneurotic edema
   d. Therapy
      i. Stop transfusion
      ii. Treat with antihistamines and/or sympathomimetics
      iii. Resume transfusion with washed red cells
5. Other complications
   a. *Volume overload*, especially dangerous in patients with cardiac disease; overload is less likely with washed packed cells
   b. *Hypothermia*, if blood is cold
   c. *$K^+$ overload* in patients with renal failure; $K^+$ concentration rises from 6 mEq/L to 21 mEq/L over 21 days of storage if blood is not frozen
   d. *Elevated ammonia levels* in patients with liver disease; ammonia concentration rises from 50 $\mu$g/dL to 700 $\mu$g/dL over 21 days of storage if blood is not frozen

## DIFFERENTIAL DIAGNOSIS OF ANEMIA: INITIAL CHARACTERIZATION

1. The diagnosis of anemia is confirmed by demonstrating a decrease in the hemoglobin concentration and hematocrit.
2. The initial step in identifying the specific etiology is to determine whether the disorder is one of underproduction (hypoproliferative) or destruction (hemolytic). This distinction can be made by obtaining a reticulocyte count.
3. If the anemia is hypoproliferative, determination of red blood cell indices (mean corpuscular volume [MCV] and mean corpuscular hemoglobin [MCH]) will allow further subcategorization.
4. If the anemia is hemolytic, a Coombs test will reveal whether the hemolysis is immunologic or nonimmunologic
5. The causes of anemia can thus be grossly subdivided as follows:
    a. Hypoproliferative (low or normal reticulocyte count)
        i. Macrocytic (increased mean corpuscular volume)
        ii. Normochromic, normocytic (normal indices)
        iii. Microcytic, hypochromic (decreased mean corpuscular volume and mean corpuscular hemoglobin)
    b. Hemolytic (increased reticulocyte count)
        i. Immune (Coombs positive)
        ii. Nonimmune (Coombs negative)

## MACROCYTIC ANEMIA: DIFFERENTIAL DIAGNOSIS

A bone marrow examination will reveal whether the cells of the erythroblast series are enlarged (megaloblastic) or not. In megaloblastic anemia, enlarged red blood cells and hypersegmented polymophonuclear leucocytes can be seen in the peripheral blood.

1. Nonmegaloblastic
   a. Alcoholism (if not associated with folate deficiency)
   b. Liver disease
   c. Hypothyroidism
2. Megaloblastic
   a. Vitamin $B_{12}$ deficiency
      i. Loss of intrinsic factor: pernicious anemia, gastrectomy
      ii. Competition for vitamin $B_{12}$: bacterial overgrowth (blind loops, diverticula, mechanical abnormalities, enterocolic contamination, prolonged antibiotic therapy)
      iii. Impaired absorption: inflammatory bowel disease, ileal resection
      iv. Dietary deficiency (rare)
   b. Folate deficiency
      i. Drugs: phenytoin, folate antagonists
      ii. Malabsorption
      iii. Dietary deficiency (most common): alcoholism (most common setting)

### Vitamin $B_{12}$ vs. Folate Deficiency

| $B_{12}$ | Folate |
|---|---|
| Neurologic symptoms | No neurologic symptoms |
|   Altered cerebration | |
|   Subacute combined degeneration | |
| Laboratory | |
|   Decreased serum $B_{12}$ | Normal |
|   Increased urinary methylmalonic acid | Normal |
|   Normal serum folate | Decreased |

## NORMOCHROMIC, NORMOCYTIC ANEMIA: DIFFERENTIAL DIAGNOSIS

1. Anemia of chronic disease
   a. Chronic inflammation or infection
   b. Neoplastic disease
   c. Uremia
2. Marrow aplasia
   a. Aplastic anemia
      i. Drugs (especially chloramphenicol and cancer chemotherapy)
      ii. Toxins (especially benzene, toluene, insecticides, carbon tetrachloride)
      iii. Infiltration (leukemia, myelofibrosis)
   b. Pure red cell aplasia
3. Early iron deficiency

## MICROCYTIC, HYPOCHROMIC ANEMIA: DIFFERENTIAL DIAGNOSIS

| | Bone marrow | Transferrin saturation | Ferritin | Additional comments |
|---|---|---|---|---|
| Iron deficiency<br>Dietary deficiency or blood loss (esp. menstruating females) | Iron stores are absent | Decreased | Decreased | — |
| Thalassemia | Normal | Normal or increased | Normal or increased | Definitive test is hemoglobin electrophoresis |
| Anemia of chronic disease | Normal or increased iron stores | Normal | Normal | Anemia is usually mild |
| Sideroblastic anemia<br>Inherited<br>Drug-induced (esp. alcohol, chloramphenicol, isoniazid)<br>Lead poisoning | Ringed sideroblasts | Normal or increased | Increased | — |

# HEMOLYTIC ANEMIAS:
## DIFFERENTIAL DIAGNOSIS

1. Coombs Positive
   a. Transfusion reactions
   b. Autoimmune
      i. Idiopathic
      ii. Associated with an underlying illness (lymphoproliferative disorders, infections, inflammatory disorders)
      iii. Drug-related (including penicillin, quinidine, quinine, methyldopa, sulfonamides, cephalosporins, isoniazid, rifampicin)
      iv. Cold agglutinins: idiopathic, associated with an underlying illness (as above), paroxysmal nocturnal hemogloblinuria
2. Coombs Negative
   a. Mechanical hemolysis
      i. Prosthetic valves
      ii. Malignant hypertension
      iii. Disseminated intravascular coagulation (DIC)
   b. Sickle cell anemia
   c. Glucose-6-phosphate dehydrogenase deficiency
   d. Hereditary membrane disorders (e.g., spherocytosis, elliptocytosis)
   e. Associated with underlying disease (hepatic, renal, infectious—especially malaria, brucellosis, and infectious endocarditis)

## CAUSES OF SPLENOMEGALY

1. Neoplastic disease
   a. Lymphoma
   b. Leukemia (especially dramatic in CML, myelofibrosis, and hairy cell leukemia)
   c. Metastatic disease
2. Infection
   a. Viral: mononucleosis, CMV, hepatitis
   b. Bacterial: TB, endocarditis, brucellosis, syphilis, typhoid
   c. Fungal: histoplasmosis
   d. Parasitic: toxoplasmosis, malaria
   e. Rickettsial: Rocky Mountain Spotted Fever
3. Infiltrative disease
   a. Sarcoidosis
   b. Amyloidosis
   c. Lipid storage diseases
4. Immunologic–inflammatory diseases
   a. Systemic lupus erythematosus (SLE)
   b. Felty's syndrome
   c. Idiopathic thrombocytopenic purpura (ITP)
5. Portal hypertension
   a. Cirrhosis of the liver
   b. Obstruction of portal or splenic veins
   c. Congestive heart failure
6. Sequestration
   a. Hemolytic anemias
   b. Spherocytosis
   c. Sickle cell disease
   d. Thalassemia

## THE COAGULATION FACTORS

| Factor | Synonym | Biologic Half-life | Vitamin K required for synthesis | Replacement therapy | Comments |
|---|---|---|---|---|---|
| *Intrinsic Pathway* | | | | | |
| VIII | Antihemophilic factor | 9–18 h | No | Cryoprecipitate or fresh frozen plasma | Hemophilia A—sex-linked recessive; von Willebrand's disease —autosomal dominant |
| IX | Christmas factor | 20–30 h | Yes | Fresh frozen plasma or concentrate | Hemophilia B—sex-linked recessive |
| XI | Plasma thromboplastin antecedent factor | 1.5–3 days | No | Fresh frozen plasma | |
| XII | Hageman factor | 2–2.5 days | No | Fresh frozen plasma | |
| *Extrinsic Pathway* | | | | | |
| VII | Proconvertin | 2–6 h | Yes | Fresh frozen plasma or concentrate | Shortest half-life, therefore deficiency is earliest evidence of vitamin K deficiency |

*Common Pathway*

| | | | |
|---|---|---|---|
| I | Fibrinogen | 3–5 days | No | Cryoprecipitate |
| II | Prothrombin | 2–4 days | Yes | Fresh frozen plasma or concentrate |
| V | Proaccelerin | 12–36 h | No | Fresh frozen plasma |
| X | Stuart-Prower | 1–2 days | Yes | Fresh frozen plasma or concentrate |
| XIII | Fibrin stabiliz-ing factor | 4–12 days | No | Fresh frozen plasma |

## The Coagulation Cascade

The culmination of the coagulation cascade is the generation of fibrin from fibrinogen. This step requires the production of thrombin from prothrombin, which in turn requires the generation of activated factor X (Xa). Activated factor X can be generated by:

1. The *intrinsic pathway*, a cascade of reactions involving several factors and initiated by exposure of factor XII to surface factors, or
2. The *extrinsic pathway*, involving only factor VII.

*(continued)*

# THE COAGULATION FACTORS (cont.)

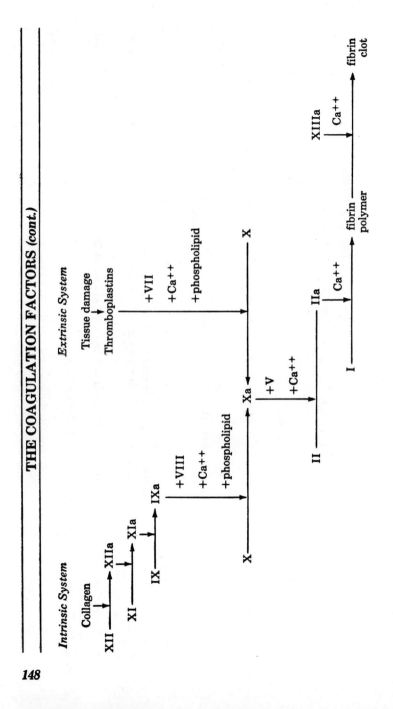

*Intrinsic System*

XII $\xrightarrow{\text{Collagen}}$ XIIa

XI $\xrightarrow{}$ XIa

IX $\xrightarrow{}$ IXa

X $\xrightarrow[\substack{+\text{VIII} \\ +\text{Ca}^{++} \\ +\text{phospholipid}}]{}$ Xa

*Extrinsic System*

$\xrightarrow[\substack{+\text{VII} \\ +\text{Ca}^{++} \\ +\text{phospholipid}}]{\substack{\text{Tissue damage} \\ \text{Thromboplastins}}}$ X

Xa $\xrightarrow[\substack{+\text{V} \\ +\text{Ca}^{++}}]{}$

II $\xrightarrow{}$ IIa

I $\xrightarrow[\text{Ca}^{++}]{}$ fibrin polymer $\xrightarrow[\text{Ca}^{++}]{\text{XIIIa}}$ fibrin clot

## COMMONLY USED TESTS OF COAGULATION

Despite the great number of available tests, a partial thromboplastin time, prothrombin time, platelet count, and bleeding time will detect the vast majority of bleeding disorders.

1. *Partial Thromboplastin Time (PTT)*: Measures clot formation via the intrinsic pathway, and therefore tests for all factors except factor VII. Cephalin and calcium chloride are added to citrated plasma and the time required for clot formation is noted (normal, 30–45 seconds). It is the best single test to screen for a disorder or deficiency of a coagulation factor.

2. *Prothrombin Time (PT)*: Measures clot formation via the extrinsic pathway, and therefore tests for factors VII, X, V, II, and I. Thromboplastin and calcium are added to plasma and the time to clot formation is recorded (normal 12–15 seconds). It is an excellent screen for vitamin K deficiency and is used to monitor patients on long-term anticoagulant therapy.

3. *Platelet Count:* Can be done quantitatively (normal 150,000–400,000 mm$^2$) or simply by examining a blood film. Because thrombocytopenia is by far the most common cause of platelet-related bleeding, an examination of a peripheral blood film is a useful and easy screen for a platelet dyscrasia.

4. *Bleeding Time:* Measures the time for a standardized incision to stop bleeding (normal 2–7 minutes). In a patient with a normal PTT, PT, and platelet count, a prolonged bleeding time suggests a disorder of platelet function or, less commonly, a vascular defect.

## THE USE OF ANTICOAGULANTS

|  | *Heparin* | *Warfarin* |
|---|---|---|
| Mechanism of action | Potentiates the action of antithrombin III, which inhibits the activity of thrombin and several activated clotting factors | Inhibits vitamin K-dependent synthesis of factors II, VII, IX, X |
| Metabolism | Metabolized by liver, inactive metabolites excreted in urine | Heavily bound to albumin, metabolized by liver, inactive metabolites excreted in urine and stool |
| Best index of efficiency of anticoagulation | PTT | PT |
| Mode of administration | IV, subcutaneous | Oral |
| Antidote | Protamine sulfate | Vitamin K or a transfusion containing vitamin K-dependent factors (e.g., fresh frozen plasma) |
| Major side effects | Hemorrhage, thrombocytopenia (usually transient and mild) | Hemorrhage |
| Less common side effects | Allergic reactions, osteoporosis, chest pain, hypotension, alopecia, hyponatremia | Thrombocytopenia, rash, fever, nausea, vomiting, diarrhea, jaundice, vasculitis, alopecia, leukopenia, nephropathy |

## Contraindications to Anticoagulation

1. Active bleeding (e.g., from a peptic ulcer)
2. Bleeding diathesis (e.g., hemophilia)
3. Intracranial hemorrhage
4. Severe hypertension
5. Infectious endocarditis
6. Active tuberculosis
7. Patients undergoing a lumbar puncture or surgery of the eye or CNS
8. Pregnancy (warfarin only; warfarin crosses the placenta and can cause fatal hemorrhage)

## COMMON DRUGS THAT INTERACT WITH COUMARIN COMPOUNDS

1. *Drugs that potentiate anticoagulant effects*
   a. Antipyretic and anti-inflammatory agents (indomethacin, phenylbutazone, and salicylates in large doses)
   b. Anabolic steroids
   c. Antilipemic agents (clofibrate and D-thyroxine)
   d. Sulfonamide antibiotics
   e. Quinidine and quinine
   f. Disulfiram
2. *Drugs that diminish anticoagulant effects*
   a. Ethanol
   b. Barbiturates
   c. Glutethimide
   d. Griseofulvin
   e. Mercurial diuretics
   f. Rifampin
   g. Cholestyramine

# THROMBOCYTOPENIA: DIFFERENTIAL DIAGNOSIS

1. *Decreased platelet production*
   a. Drug toxicity (especially alcohol and thiazide diuretics)
   b. Radiation to marrow
   c. Marrow replacement (leukemia, myelofibrosis)
   d. Aplastic anemia
   e. Vitamin $B_{12}$ or folate deficiency
   f. Uremia
   g. Sepsis

2. *Increased platelet destruction*
   a. Drug toxicity (especially quinidine and quinine, also sulfonamides, para-aminosalicylic acid, heparin, gold, methyldopa)
   b. ITP
   c. TTP
   d. DIC

3. *Abnormal distribution*
   a. Splenomegaly (causing sequestration)

## DIFFERENCES IN PLATELET AND COAGULATION
## FACTOR DISORDERS

|  | *Platelet disorder (usually thrombocytopenia)* | *Coagulation factor disorder* |
|---|---|---|
| Most characteristic type of bleeding | Petechiae in the skin and mucous membranes due to bleeding from superficial small vessels | Deep tissue bleeding, especially in muscles and joints, occurring spontaneously or after minor trauma |

*Screening tests*

| | | |
|---|---|---|
| PT | Normal | Normal or increased |
| PTT | Normal | Increased in approximately 90% of patients |
| Platelet count | Usually decreased | Normal |
| Bleeding time | Usually prolonged | Usually normal, occasionally prolonged |
| Predisposition | Females > males | Males > females |
| Family history | Family history often negative | Family history often positive |
| Treatment | Platelet concentrates | Fresh frozen plasma or specific factor concentrates |

## PLATELET DYSFUNCTION: COMMON DRUGS THAT INTERACT WITH PLATELETS AND PROLONG BLEEDING TIME

1. Anti-inflammatory agents
   a. Aspirin
   b. Phenylbutazone
   c. Sulfinpyrazone
2. Antihistamines: diphenhydramine (Benadryl)
3. Phenothiazines
   a. Chlorpromazine
   b. Promethazine
4. Tricyclic antidepressants
   a. Imipramine (Tofranil)
   b. Amitryptyline (Elavil)
5. Dextran
6. Dipyridamole (Persantine)

## DISSEMINATED INTRAVASCULAR COAGULATION (DIC)

1. Most common etiologies
   a. Infection: severe sepsis, generally gram negative
   b. Liberation of tissue factors into the circulation
      i. Massive hemolysis (e.g., acute transfusion reactions)
      ii. Obstetric catastrophes
      iii. Fat emboli
      iv. Tumors (especially prostatic cancer and acute promyelocytic leukemia)
   c. Endothelial injury
      i. Severe hypotension and shock
      ii. Heatstroke
      iii. Burns
      iv. Immune complex disease (e.g., acute glomerulonephritis)
      v. Rocky Mountain Spotted Fever
2. Characteristic laboratory findings
   a. Microangiopathic hemolysis (red cell fragments on a blood film)
   b. Anemia
   c. Increased fibrin split products
   d. Prolonged PT and PTT
   e. Decreased platelet count
   f. Decreased fibrinogen

## POLYCYTHEMIA: DIFFERENTIAL DIAGNOSIS

1. Primary erythrocytosis
   a. Polycythemia vera (PCV)
2. Hypoxia-stimulating erythropoietin production
   a. Pulmonary disease
      i. Chronic obstructive lung disease
      ii. Interstitial fibrosis
      iii. Lung cancer
      iv. High altitude
   b. Cardiac disease: right-to-left shunts
   c. Mechanical disorder: obesity (including Pickwickian syndrome)
   d. Abnormal hemoglobins
3. Tumors that produce erythropoietin
   a. Renal tumors
      i. Hypernephroma
      ii. Renal adenoma
      iii. Undifferentiated renal carcinoma
   b. Hepatoma
   c. Cerebellar hemangioblastoma
   d. Pheochromocytoma
   e. Uterine fibromyoma
4. Other causes
   a. Renal disease
      i. Cysts
      ii. Hydronephrosis
   b. Cushing's syndrome
   c. Stress erythrocytosis (Gaisbock's syndrome): relative polycythemia due to hemoconcentration, diuretic therapy, or prolonged diarrhea, or idiopathic.

## COMPLICATIONS OF LEUKEMIA

1. Infection: Infection is the leading cause of death in acute leukemia, and is due to immunosuppression resulting from the disease itself, cachexia, and chemotherapeutic drugs. Gram negative organisms are seen most commonly, but gram positive bacteria, fungi, toxoplasma, and pneumocystis are also encountered.
2. Hemorrhage: Hemorrhage is the second leading cause of death in leukemia, and is usually due to thrombocytopenia. In 10% of patients, DIC is the cause. Intracerebral bleeding poses the greatest danger to the patient, but gastrointestinal and pulmonary hemorrhages may also be fatal.
3. Anemia: Anemia is common, occurring in the vast majority of patients, and transfusions are often required.
4. Hyperviscosity: Hyperviscosity results from the massive numbers of leucocytes in the circulation, and can lead to blurred vision, weakness, abdominal pain, congestive heart failure, and stroke.
5. Hypokalemia: Hypokalemia is especially prevalent in AML.
6. Hyperkalemia: Hyperkalemia usually occurs during chemotherapy, when the resultant massive cell death leads to the release of intracellular potassium stores.
7. Hyperuricemia: Hyperuricemia results from the turnover of malignant cells, and is therefore also common during chemotherapy. Uric acid nephropathy can result, and most patients are therefore given allopurinol prophylactically.

## HISTOLOGIC CLASSIFICATION OF MALIGNANT LYMPHOMAS

| *Disorder* | *Prognostic features* |
|---|---|
| Hodgkin's disease<br>  Lymphocyte predominance<br>  Mixed cellularity<br>  Lymphocyte depletion<br>  Nodular sclerosis | Prognosis worsens as the number of lymphocytes decreases |
| Non-Hodgkin's lymphomas<br>  Lymphocytic lymphoma<br>    Well differentiated, nodular<br>    Poorly differentiated, nodular<br>    Poorly differentiated, diffuse<br>  Histiocytic lymphoma<br>    Nodular<br>    Diffuse<br>  Mixed histiocytic–lymphocytic<br>  lymphoma<br>  Undifferentiated lymphoma<br>    Burkitt's<br>    non-Burkitt's | Nodular lymphomas carry a better prognosis than diffuse lymphomas |

## STAGING CLASSIFICATION FOR
## MALIGNANT LYMPHOMAS

Stage I: Involvement of a single lymph node region (I) or of a single extralymphatic site (IE).

Stage II: Involvment of two or more lymph node regions on the same side of the diaphragm (II) or localized involvement of a single extralymphatic site plus one or more lymph node regions on the same side of the diaphragm (IIE).

Stage III: Involvement of lymph node regions on both sides of the diaphragm (III), which may be accompanied by involvement of an extralymphatic site (IIIE), the spleen (IIIS), or both (IIISE).

Stage IV: Disseminated involvement of one or more extralymphatic sites with or without lymph node involvement.

A letter classification is also assigned depending upon whether there are:

A. No systemic symptoms, or
B. Fever, night sweats, or weight loss exceeding 10% of body weight

## STAGING PROCEDURES FOR MALIGNANT LYMPHOMA

1. History and physical examination.
2. Liver function tests.
3. Chest x-ray and metastatic bone survey.
4. Bone marrow examination.
5. Liver–spleen scan.
6. Lower extremity lymphangiograms.
7. Lymph node biopsies.
8. Laparotomy, with sampling of nodes and liver and a splenectomy (laparotomy with splenectomy is usually omitted in patients with non-Hodgkin's lymphoma, since the disease is almost always detected in stages III and IV and radiation therapy can be of little value).*
9. Abdominal CT scan.

*Additional chemistries and radiologic procedures may precede laparotomy in the hope of detecting diffuse spread without the necessity of surgery.

# Section

# 5

# Rheumatology

## SYNOVIAL FLUID ANALYSIS

The following tests should be performed on a patient with un-diagnosed joint disease and a joint effusion. Aspirate the effusion into a sterile heparinized syringe and divide into four tubes.

### Tube one (plain)

1. Determination of fluid volume
2. Assessment of gross appearance, noting:
   a. Color
   b. Clarity, measured by attempting to read print through the fluid contained in glass (not plastic)
   c. Viscosity, measured by watching the fluid emerge from a syringe tip.
3. A mucin clot test, performed by adding a few drops of synovial fluid to 20 mL of 5% acetic acid. The firmness of the resultant clot is a measure of the mucopolysarcharide content of the effusion

### Tube two (anticoagulated, not oxalate)

4. Microscopic examination
   a. Cell count and differential (Wright's stain)
   b. Gram stain and, if indicated, Ziehl-Neelsen stain for tuberculosis
   c. Crystal identification: only the presence of crystals *within* cells (neutrophils) can confirm the diagnosis of gout or pseudogout. Polarimetry can also be helpful

### Tube three (plain, sterile)

5. Culture for aerobic and anaerobic organisms, tuberculosis, and fungi. Thayer-Martin medium under $CO_2$ may be required to isolate gonococci

### Tube four (anticoagulated, not oxalate)

6. Chemistries: glucose levels decline in the presence of large numbers of cells or, especially, microorganisms
7. Immunologic tests include:
   a. Complement level (compared with serum level)
   b. Antinuclear antibodies
   c. Hepatitis B antigen
   d. LE cell test
   e. Latex fixation for rheumatoid factor
   f. Search for RA cells

## CLASSIFICATION OF JOINT FLUID

Analyzing synovial fluid aspirated from an affected joint can suggest the cause of an effusion.

1. The presence of a small effusion (3.5 mL) does not guarantee the absence of significant joint disease.
2. Streaks of blood indicate injury to a small vessel during aspiration.

### Examination of Joint Fluid

| Measure | Normal | Group I (Noninflammatory) | Group II (Inflammatory) | Group III (Septic) |
|---|---|---|---|---|
| Volume (mL) | <3.5 | Often >3.5 | Often >3.5 | Often >3.5 |
| Appearance | Clear and colorless | Clear and straw-colored | Translucent and yellow | Opaque |
| Viscosity | High | High | Low | Variable |
| WBC (per mm³) | <200 | 200 to 2,000 | 2,000 to 100,000 | >1,000,000* |
| Polymorphonuclear leucocytes (%) | <25% | <25% | 50% or more (containing crystals in gout and pseudogout) | 75% or more* |
| Gram stain | No organisms | No organisms | No organisms | Organisms often present |
| Culture | Negative | Negative | Negative | Often positive |
| Mucin clot | Firm | Firm | Friable | Friable |
| Glucose (mg/100 mL) | Nearly equal to blood | Nearly equal to blood | >25, lower than blood | <25, much lower than blood |
| Crystals | None | None | Present in gout and pseudogout | None |

*Lower with infections caused by partially treated or low-virulence organisms.

## DIFFERENTIAL DIAGNOSIS OF JOINT DISEASE ACCORDING TO JOINT FLUID CLASSIFICATION

### Noninflammatory: Characteristic Clinical Findings

1. Degenerative joint disease: DIP (Heberden's nodes) and PIP (Bouchard's nodes) involved; MCP and wrist joints spared; no signs of inflammation; pain worse with activity
2. Traumatic arthritis: evidence and history of trauma
3. Hypertrophic pulmonary osteoarthropathy: clubbing of fingers
4. Early rheumatoid arthritis: early involvement of hands (PIP, MCP) with swelling, warmth, tenderness, morning stiffness and pain prodrome of weakness, fatigue, aches
5. Others
   a. Amyloidosis
   b. Acromegaly
   c. Neuropathic arthropathy
   d. Osteochondritis dissecans
   e. Hemachromatosis
   f. Villonodular synovitis
   g. Sickle cell disease
   h. Wilson's disease
   i. Pancreatitis
   j. Resolving inflammatory arthritis

### Inflammatory: Characteristic Clinical Findings

1. Polyarticular, primarily peripheral joint involvement
   a. Rheumatoid arthritis: symmetric, not migratory; PIP, MCP, wrist involvement; subcutaneous nodules
   b. Juvenile rheumatoid arthritis: onset before age 16; subcutaneous nodules are rare; may have associated rash, serositis, lymphadenopathy, splenomegaly
   c. Rheumatic fever: migratory; primarily affects large joints; affects children, young adults; history of streptococcal infection
   d. Connective tissue diseases (SLE, polymyositis, PSS, MCTD): joint involvement is rarely severe, does not lead to deformity; females predominate; systemic signs and symptoms
   e. Polyarteritis nodosa: migratory; joints rarely involved severely; nodular lesions on skin, mucous membranes
   f. Sarcoidosis: lower extremities primarily involved, often early in course
   g. Serum sickness: migratory; large and small joints involved; rash is common; history of penicillin, horse serum, or other drug administration

2. Monoarticular involvement

True monoarticular diseases are characterized by the rapid onset of pain and swelling, and by the appearance of a joint effusion and periarticular erythema. The last virtually rules out the possibility of a polyarticular disease masquerading as a monoarticular arthritis.

    a. Gout: tophi, podagra; intense inflammatory attacks; look for precipitating factors (drugs, trauma, etc.)

    b. Pseudogout: acute attacks resemble gout, but predilection for larger joints, especially knee

    c. Viral arthritis (especially rubella and hepatitis): history of local epidemic; spontaneous remission

3. Polyarthritis with vertebral involvement

    a. Reiter's syndrome: asymmetric peripheral involvement; spine involvement also asymmetric; associated urethritis and conjunctivitis; varied skin involvement; primarily affects young men

    b. Ankylosing spondylitis: hip and shoulder involvement; spinal inflammation progresses to fusion; young males primarily affected

    c. Psoriatic arthritis: asymmetric DIP involvement is virtually pathognomonic; spine involvement indistinguishable from Reiter's syndrome; skin and nail lesions

    d. Inflammatory bowel disease: predilection for large joints

4. Other, less common causes of arthritis

    a. Infectious (fungal, parasitic, mycoplasmal, tuberculous)

    b. Vasculitis (polymyalgia rheumatica, Wegener's granulomatosis, giant cell arteritis, Henoch-Schonlein purpura)

    c. Whipple's disscase

    d. Familial Mediterranean Fever

    e. Bacterial endocarditis

## Septic: Characteristic Clinical Findings

1. Bacterial infections: acute onset; fever, chills, primarily affect large joints, especially the knee

    a. Gonococcal arthritis: initially polyarticular, often migratory, then localizes in 1 or 2 joints; may have skin lesions or genitourinary complaints; history of exposure

    b. *Staphylococcus aureus:* history of underlying rheumatoid arthritis is common

    c. Much less common: *Streptococcus pneumoniae; H. influenzae* flu and other gram negative organisms; tuberculosis

## DIFFERENTIAL DIAGNOSIS OF JOINT DISEASE ACCORDING TO JOINT FLUID CLASSIFICATION *(cont.)*

### Hemorrhagic

1. Trauma
2. Bleeding diathesis (e.g., hemophilia, anticoagulation therapy)
3. Neuropathic arthropathy
4. Villonodular synovitis
5. Synovial hemangoima

## GOUT VERSUS PSEUDOGOUT

### Crystal Identification

| | *Chemical composition* | *Microscopic appearance* | *Polarimetry with 1st order red compensator* | *Therapy* |
|---|---|---|---|---|
| Gout | Monosodium urate | Thin and needle-like | Crystals exhibit negative birefringence, appearing yellow when aligned parallel to the compensator axis | *Acute attack:* Colchicine-IV dose has less GI side effects than oral dose (pain, nausea, vomiting, diarrhea) *Chronic maintenance:* Overproducers of uric acid should receive allopurinol, adjusted to keep the uric acid level normal. Underexcretors of uric acid should receive a uricosuric (probenecid, sulfinpyrazone) |
| Pseudogout | Calcium pyrophosphate | Pleomorphic, blunt and rectangular | Crystals show weak, positive birefringence, appearing blue when parallel to the compensator axis | A brief course of a nonsteroidal anti-inflammatory agent, such as phenylbutazone or indomethacin, will usually abort an acute attack |

# Section

# 6

# Fluids and Electrolytes

# ELECTROLYTE CONTENT OF SWEAT AND GI SECRETIONS

**Electrolyte concentration, mEq/L**

| | $Na^+$ | $K^+$ | $H^+$ | $Cl^-$ | $HCO_3^-$ |
|---|---|---|---|---|---|
| Sweat | 50 | 5 | – | 55 | – |
| Gastric secretions | 40 | 10 | 90 | 140 | – |
| Pancreatic fluid | 135 | 5 | – | 50 | 90 |
| Bile | 135 | 5 | – | 105 | 35 |
| Small-intestine fluid | 130 | 10 | – | 115 | 25 |
| Diarrheal fluid | 50 | 35 | – | 40 | 45 |

**Replace each liter lost with**

| | *Normal Saline (ml)* | *D5W (ml)* | *KCl (mEq)* | *$NaHCO_3$ (mEq)* |
|---|---|---|---|---|
| Sweat | 300 | 700 | 5 | – |
| Gastric secretions | 250 | 750 | 20* | – |
| Pancreatic fluid | 250 | 750 | 5 | 90† |
| Bile | 750 | 250 | 5 | 45 |
| Small-intestine fluid | 750 | 250 | 10 | 22 |
| Diarrheal fluid | – | 1000 | 35 | 45 |

Adapted from Freitag JJ, Miller LW: Manual of Medical Therapeutics, 23rd ed. Little, Brown and Company, Boston, 1980, p. 26.

*Excess potassium is often required because of increased urinary potassium excretion in alkalosis.

†One ampule of 7.5% $NaHCo_3$ contains 45mEq $HCO_3$.

## UNCOMPLICATED ACID-BASE DISORDERS

| Disorder | PH | PCO₂ | (HCO₃⁻) |
|---|---|---|---|
| Metabolic acidosis | Decreased | Decreased | Decreased |
| Metabolic alkalosis | Increased | Increased | Increased |
| Respiratory acidosis | Decreased | Increased | Increased |
| Respiratory alkalosis | Increased | Decreased | Decreased |

$$pH = 6.1 + \frac{[HCO_3^-]}{\log .03 \times Paco_2}$$

1. Signs of *acidosis* may include
   a. Kussmaul respirations
   b. Restlessness
   c. Disorientation
   d. Hypotension
2. Signs of *alkalosis* may include
   a. Paresthesias
   b. Weakness
   c. Tetany
   d. Convulsions

## METABOLIC ACIDOSIS: DIFFERENTIAL DIAGNOSIS

Calculation of the anion gap: $[Na^+] - ([Cl^-] + [HCO_3^-]) =$ anion gap; normal gap is 8–12

1. *Normal anion gap (i.e., loss of bicarbonate; associated with hyperchloremia)*
   a. Diarrhea
   b. Pancreatic fistula
   c. Ureterosigmoidostomy
   d. Drugs
      i. Acidifying agents
      ii. Carbonic anhydrase inhibitors (e.g., acetazolamide)
      iii. Cholestyramine
   e. Interstitial renal disease
   f. Renal tubular acidosis
   g. Hyperalimentation with chloride salts
2. *Increased anion gap*
   a. Toxic ingestions (i.e., addition of a strong acid)
      i. Salicylates
      ii. Methanol
      iii. Ethylene glycol
      iv. Paraldehyde
   b. Acid retention
      i. Diabetic ketoacidosis
      ii. Uremia
      iii. Starvation
      iv. Lactic acidosis (e.g., from shock, hypoxia, DKA, phenformin, or occasionally, idiopathic)
      v. Alcoholic acidosis

## RENAL TUBULAR ACIDOSIS

1. Type 1: Distal renal tubular acidosis
   a. Pathophysiology: failure of distal tubule to secrete $H^+$ ions
   b. Urine pH: greater than 5.5
   c. Serum $HCO_3^-$: less than 15 mEq/L
   d. Etiology
      i. Primary
      ii. Nephrocalcinosis of any cause (including hyperparathyroidism, vitamin D intoxication, medullary sponge kidney, and idiopathic hypercalciuria)
      iii. Hypergammaglobulinemic disorders (including myeloma, cryoglobulinemia, and most autoimmune diseases)
      iv. Drug toxicity: amphotericin B, toluene, lithium
      v. Hepatic cirrhosis
      vi. Pyelonephritis and obstructive uropathy
      vii. Sickle-cell anemia
2. Type 2: Proximal renal tubular acidosis
   a. Pathophysiology: failure of proximal tubule to resorb bicarbonate
   b. Urine pH: 4.8–5.5 (approximately normal)
   c. Serum $HCO_3^-$: greater than 15 mEq/L
   d. Etiology
      i. Primary (part of Fanconi's syndrome)
      ii. Hyperparathyroidism
      iii. Myeloma and amyloidosis
      iv. Heavy metals
      v. Nephrotic syndrome
      vi. Sjögren's syndrome
      vii. Ingestion of outdated tetracycline
      viii. Following renal transplantation
      ix. Genetic disorders (including Wilson's disease and cystinosis)

## METABOLIC ALKALOSIS:
## DIFFERENTIAL DIAGNOSIS

1. *Contraction alkalosis (chloride responsive)*
   a. Vomiting
   b. Gastric suction
   c. Diuretics (thiazides, mercurials, ethacrynic acid, furosemide)
   d. Villous adenoma of colon
   e. Relief of chronic hypercapnia
2. *Chloride resistant*
   a. Hypokalemia (severe—$K^+$ less than 2.0 mEq/L)
   b. Excessive mineralocorticoid activity
      i. Hyperaldosteronism
      ii. Cushing's syndrome
   c. Milk–alkali syndrome

## RESPIRATORY ACIDOSIS

**Causes:**

*Acute*

General anesthesia
Sedative overdosage
Cardiac arrest
Pneumothorax
Pulmonary edema
Severe pneumonia
Bronchospasm or laryngospasm
Foreign body aspiration
Mechanical ventilators

*Chronic*

Obstructive pulmonary
  disease
Primary alveolar hypo-
  ventilation
Neuromuscular disorder (e.g.,
  polio, myopathies)
Restrictive disease of thorax
  (kyphoscoliosis)

**Concurrent acid-base disturbances:**

An increase of 10 mmHG of $PaCO_2$ causes an increase in $[HCO_3^-]$ (plasma) by 1 mEq/L

If the increase in $[HCO_3^-]$ is < 1 mEq/L, then there is a coexisting metabolic acidosis, commonly due to renal insufficiency or tissue hypoxia with lactic acidosis

If the increase in $[HCO_3^-]$ is > 3 mEq/L, then there is a coexisting metabolic alkalosis, commonly due to use of a respirator (with rapid decrease of $PCO_2$, there is a persisting elevation of $[HCO3_-]$), hypochloremia (causing increased renal bicarbonate reabsorption), hypokalemia (causing increased renal $H^+$ loss), and diuretics (causing increased $Na^+$ delivery to the distal tubules and increased $H^+$ excretion)

## RESPIRATORY ALKALOSIS

### Causes

1. Known mechanisms:
   a. Hypoxemic stimulation of peripheral chemoreceptors
   b. Distention of pulmonary vascular tree
   c. Stimulation of midbrain respiratory centers (lesions, drugs, endotoxins) or increased intracranial pressures
   d. Improper regulation of ventilators

2. Common disorders:
   a. Anxiety, hysteria
   b. Fever
   c. Salicylate intoxication
   d. Cerebrovascular accident
   e. Congestive heart failure
   f. Pneumonia
   g. Pulmonary emboli
   h. Hypoxia
   i. Hepatic insufficiency
   j. Gram-negative sepsis

### Concomitant disorders:

Acutely: For each decrease of 10 mm Hg in $PaCO_2$, there is a fall in $[HCO_3^-]$ (plasma) of approximately 1.5 mEq/L (increased lactate generation)

Chronic: For each decrease of 10 mm Hg in $PaCO_2$, there is a fall in $[HCO_3^-]$ (plasma of approximately 3.0 mEq/L (decreased $H^+$ excretion)

If the decrease in $[HCO_3^-]$ (plasma) is greater than expected, suspect concomitant superimposed metabolic alkalosis.

## CAUSES OF LACTIC ACIDOSIS

### Overproduction of Lactate

Increased oxygen requirements
  Exercise
  Generalized seizures
  Hypoxic tissue (ischemic or infarcting tissue, especially bowel)
Decreased oxygen supply to tissue
  Hypotension or shock
  Cardiac arrest
  Pulmonary disorder (neuromuscular or parenchymal) causing
    severe hypoxemia
Interference with oxygen utilization ("dysoxia")
  Phenformin
  INH overdosage
  CO poisoning
Increased glycolysis
  Diabetes mellitus, primarily with ketoacidosis
  Leukemias, lymphomas, visceral metastatic disease
  Other chronic diseases

### Decreased Utilization of Lactate

Hepatic failure (decreased perfusion, hepatocyte failure)
Ethanol intoxication

### Factitious Lactic Acidosis

Prolonged storage of arterial blood gas sample at room temperature,
  especially if leukocytosis

## DEHYDRATION

1. *Signs and symptoms*
   a. Orthostatic hypotension
   b. Tachycardia
   c. Weak pulse
   d. Poor skin turgor (test over sternum or forehead)
   e. Dry mucous membrances
   f. Low jugular venous pressure
   g. Diminished axillary sweat
   h. Dry tongue with deep furrows
   i. Weight loss (often exceeding 0.2 kg/day)
   j. Apathy
   k. Weakness
2. *Laboratory*
   a. Increased hemoglobin and hematocrit
   b. Prerenal azotemia (elevated BUN and creatinine with BUN : Creatinine ratio > 15)
   c. $Na^+$ may be low, normal, or high
   d. Diminished CVP and pulmonary wedge pressures

## VOLUME OVERLOAD

1. *Signs and symptoms*
   a. Edema
   b. Hypertension
   c. Elevated jugular venous pulse
   d. Gallop rhythm $S_3$, $S_4$
   e. Weight gain
   f. Oliguria
   g. Dyspnea
2. *Laboratory*
   a. Hyponatremia is usually present
   b. CVP and pulmonary wedge pressures are usually elevated
   c. Hematocrit is normal or low

## HYPONATREMIA

### Clinical manifestations

1. Anorexia, nausea, vomiting
2. Neurologic symptoms
   a. Lethargy, confusion, coma
   b. Weakness and cramps
   c. Seizures
   d. Myoclonus

### Etiology

Hyponatremia can occur with excess, normal, or low total body water. Each is associated with a particular set of possible etiologies:

1. Overhydration
   a. Congestive heart failure
   b. Cirrhosis
   c. Nephrotic syndrome
   d. Inappropriate ADH secretion
2. Euhydration
   a. Diuretics
   b. Inappropriate ADH secretion
3. Dehydration
   a. Renal losses
      i. Diuretics
      ii. Mineralocorticoid deficiency
   b. Gastrointestinal losses
      i. Vomiting
      ii. Diarrhea
   c. Sweating

### Therapy

1. Water restriction is usually adequate in cases of hyponatremia associated with excess or normal body water.
2. Hyponatremia associated with dehydration requires replacement with hypertonic saline.

## HYPERNATREMIA

### Clinical Manifestations

1. Neurologic symptoms*
   a. Lethargy, stupor, coma
   b. Seizures
   c. Weakness
   d. Myoclonus
2. Prerenal azotemia

### Etiology

1. Failure of an obtundated patient to drink
2. Restriction of fluid in a hospitalized patient
3. Renal water wasting
   a. Diabetes insipidus (central and nephrogenic)
   b. Osmotic diuresis (diabetes mellitus, mannitol, urea)
   c. Recovery phase of acute renal failute
4. Loss of water through the skin and lungs
   a. Burns
   b. Sweat

### Therapy

1. Gradual water replacement is required

*Because thirst mechanisms ordinarily prevent hypernatremia, it is usually found only in patients who are comatose, incapacitated by a stroke, or otherwise unable to respond to thirst. The neurologic symptoms of hypernatremia may therefore be obscured by the underlying disease.

## HYPOKALEMIA

### Common Causes

1. Extracellular-to-intracellular potassium shifts
   a. Decreased blood hydrogen ion concentration (increased pH)
   b. Increased plasma bicarbonate concentration (a 10 mm Hg decrease in $PCO_2$ causes a 0.5 mEq/L decrease in serum $K^+$)
   c. Increased plasma insulin
   d. Familial hypokalemic paralysis
2. Decreased potassium intake
   a. Carbohydrate diet
   b. Alcoholism
3. Gastrointestinal losses
   a. Salivary, pancreatic, or bile fistula
   b. Vomiting
   c. Diarrhea ($[K^+] = 20 - 30$ mEq/L)
   d. Laxative or enema abuse
   e. Ureterosigmoidostomy
   f. Villous adenoma of colon or rectum
   g. GI drainage tube
4. Increased urinary losses (>40 mEq per day)
   a. Increased mineralocorticoids
      i. Excessive secretion of ACTH from the pituitary or an ectopic site
      ii. Adrenal hyperplasia or adenoma
      iii. Primary hyperaldosteronism
      iv. Some forms of secondary hyperaldosteronism: (a) renal vascular hypertension; (b) Bartter's syndrome (decreased $K^+$, metabolic alkalosis, and increased renin and aldosterone resulting from an abnormality of renal $Cl^-$ transport)
   b. Intrinsic renal disease
      i. Renal tubular acidosis
      ii. Fanconi's syndrome
      iii. After prolonged amphotericin administration
      iv. During a postobstructive or postacute tubular necrosis diuresis
      v. After transplantation

    c. Drug induced
       i. Thiazides
      ii. Loop diuretics
     iii. Carbonic anhydrase inhibitors
     iv. Intraluminal loads of nonreabsorbable anion
      v. Licorice or carbenoxolone ingestion
     vi. Birth-control pills
    d. Hypomagnesemia
5. Leukemia with lysozymuria

## Clinical Manifestations

1. Cardiac effects
    a. ECG abnormalities (flattened or inverted P and T waves, appearance of U waves)
    b. Atrial and ventricular ectopic beats
    c. Increased risk of digitalis toxicity
2. Ileus
3. Polyuria (renal concentrating defect)
4. Weakness (when severe, flaccid paralysis and respiratory arrest)

## Therapy

1. Hypokalemia is rarely emergent, and oral potassium supplementation is usually adequate
2. In an emergency, in a patient with intact renal function, IV KCl can be given, never faster than 10 mEq/L in concentrations not exceeding 30–40 mEq/L

## HYPERKALEMIA

### Common Causes

1. Pseudohyperkalemia (artifactual due to cell lysis and release of intracellular K⁺ stores in drawn sample; confirm by finding altered serum K⁺ with normal plasma K⁺)
   a. Thrombocytosis
   b. Hemolysis
   c. Leukocytosis
2. True hyperkalemia
   a. Decreased renal excretion
      i. Oliguric renal failure: (a) acute; (b) chronic
      ii. Pharmacologic blockade of potassium secretion: (a) triamterene; (b) spironolactone; (c) amiloride
      iii. Relative or absolute hypoaldosteronism: (a) hyporeninemic aldosteronism; (b) adrenal cortical insufficiency
      iv. Isolated defect in renal excretion of potassium: (a) congenital; (b) acquired
   b. Cell leak/transcellular K⁺ shifts
      i. Acidosis: (a) metabolic; (b) respiratory
      ii. Release of intracellular K⁺: (a) crush injury; (b) from red blood cells—hemolysis and internal bleeding; (c) from malignant cells after chemotherapy—lymphomas, leukemia, and myeloma; (d) succinylcholine depolarization of cell membrane; (e) acute digitalis poisoning; (f) following arginine infusion; (g) idiopathic or familial hyperkalemic episodic paralysis
   c. High K⁺ intake
      i. Oral K⁺ supplementation
      ii. Intravenous K⁺ administration; (a) rapid administration of K⁺ solutions; (b) K⁺-penicillin in high doses; (c) rapid transfusion of aged blood
   d. Increased extracellular osmolality
      i. Glucose
      ii. Mannitol
      iii. Saline

## Clinical Manifestations

1. Cardiac toxicity
   a. Progressive ECG abnormalities
      i. Peaked T wave
      ii. Prolonged PR interval
      iii. Disappearance of P wave
      iv. Merging of QRS complex and T wave
   b. Ultimately cardiac arrest
2. Neuromuscular disorders: Paresthesias and weakness that may progress to paralysis and respiratory arrest

## Therapy

1. If mild ($K^+ <$ 6.0 mEq/L), no specific therapy is required. Reduce $K^+$ intake and correct any underlying disorder.
2. If moderate ($K^+$ 6.0–7 mEq/L), use of a potassium exchange resin (e.g. Kayexalate) is usually sufficient.
3. If severe (i.e., if cardiogenic changes seen and level above 6.5–7), then IV calcium gluconate should be used to counter the cardiac toxicity; sodium bicarbonate, glucose and insulin are given to move $K^+$ back into cells. A potassium exchange resin is also employed, and dialysis may be required.

## HYPOMAGNESEMIA

1. *Clinical manifestations*
   a. Hypokalemia and hypocalcemia, with all their attendent signs and symptoms
   b. Cardiac arrhythmias, including increased risk of digitalis toxicity
   c. Weakness
   d. Anorexia, nausea
   e. Neuromuscular symptoms, including tremor and other abnormal movements progressing to seizures
   f. Mood alterations
2. *Etiology*
   a. Alcoholism
   b. Dietary deficiency
   c. Impaired absorption
      i  Malabsorption
      ii. Excessive vomiting, diarrhea, or nasogastric suction
   d. Renal loss
      i. Diuretics
      ii. Uncontrolled diabetes mellitus
      iii. Hyperaldosteronism
      iv. Renal tubular disorders
      v. Hypercalcemia
   e. Other
      i. Hyper- and hypoparathyroidism
      ii. Acute pancreatitis
      iii. Hyperthyroidism

## Therapy

1. If emergent (seizures), IV $Mg^{++}$
2. Otherwise, oral replacement is sufficient, usually in the form of magnesium oxide.

## HYPERMAGNESEMIA

1. Symptoms
   a. Paresthesias (early sign)
   b. Peripheral vasodilation (early sign)
   c. Nausea, vomiting
   d. Lethargy and weakness progressing to flaccid paralysis
   e. Hypotension
   f. Bradycardia
   g. Respiratory depression
2. Etiology
   a. Chronic renal failure (long-term mild hypermagnesemia, usually asymptomatic); may be aggravated by an increased $Mg^{++}$ load (e.g., antacids and laxatives containing $Mg^{++}$)
   b. Other causes very uncommon

## Therapy

1. Discontinue exogenous sources of $Mg^{++}$
2. If emergent (severe respiratory or cardiac depression), give IV calcium with glucose and insulin; hemodialysis should restore normal blood levels within several hours.

*Section*

# 7

# Nephrology

## CAUSES OF HEMATURIA

1. Focal renal and genitourinary lesions
   a. Stones
   b. Infection
   c. Tumors
   d. Exercise
   e. Trauma
2. Diffuse processes
   a. Glomerulonephritis, acute and chronic
      i. Postinfectious
      ii. Associated with systemic immune complex diseases (e.g., SLE)
      iii. Idiopathic
   b. Rapidly progressive glomerulonephritis
   c. Focal glomerular sclerosis
   d. Goodpasture's syndrome
   e. Schonlein-Henoch purpura
   f. Thrombotic thrombocytopenic purpura
   g. Coagulopathies
   h. Interstitial nephritis
      i. Sickle cell disease
      ii. Diabetes mellitus
      iii. Drug-induced
      iv. Heavy metals

## URINARY TRACT INFECTIONS: DIAGNOSIS

1. Symptoms
   a. Dysuria
   b. Frequency
   c. Suprapubic tenderness
   d. Flank pain
   e. Fever and chills (generally limited to upper urinary tract infections)
2. Urinalysis and culture
   a. Examination of gram-stained unspun urine: detection of any bacteria or more than one white blood cell indicates a very high likelihood of infection
   b. Urine cultures
      i. More than 100,000 bacteria (colony-forming units) per ml of a clean-voided specimen indicates an 80% chance of infection
      ii. 10,000–100,000 bacteria rarely (5%) signifies infection
3. Upper vs lower urinary tract infections
   a. Presence of fever and chills suggest pyelonephritis
   b. Antibody-coated bacteria test is usually positive only in patients with pyelonephritis (some false positives in males with prostatitis)
4. Causative organisms in pyelonephritis and cystitis
   a. *E. coli* (most common)
   b. *Klebsiella*
   c. *Proteus*
   d. *Pseudomonas*
   e. *Enterococcus*
   f. *Staphylococcus*
5. Complications of pyelonephritis: If fever persists despite several days of antibiotic therapy, consider:
   a. Antibiotic-resistant organisms
   b. Drug reaction
   c. Septicemia
   d. Renal abscess formation
   e. Urinary tract obstruction

## OBSTRUCTIVE UROPATHY

1. Signs and symptoms
   a. Flank pain (renal colic) and tenderness
   b. Evidence of infection
   c. Hematuria
   d. Dilute polyuria
   e. Increased BUN
   f. Renal failure (with complete, bilateral obstruction)
2. Differential diagnosis
   a. Nephrolithiasis
   b. Acute uric acid nephropathy (e.g., from cytotoxic therapy)
   c. Papillary necrosis (diabetes mellitus, sickle cell disease, analgesic abuse)
   d. Carcinoma of renal pelvis or ureter
   e. Ureteral blood clot
   f. Ureteropelvic stricture or valve
   g. Bladder tumor
   h. Neurogenic bladder (diabetes mellitus)
   i. Urethral stricture or valve
   j. Genitourinary tuberculosis
   k. Prostatic obstruction (hypertrophy, inflammation, neoplasia)
   l. Carcinoma of the cervix
   m. Endometriosis
   n. Pregnancy
   o. Pelvic or retroperitoneal tumors
   p. Pelvic inflammatory disease
   q. Pelvic adhesions (radiation, surgery)
   r. Inflammatory bowel disease
   s. Aortic aneurysm

## RENAL STONES

### Calcium stones

1. Calcium oxalate or calcium phosphate (or mixed)
2. Most common type of stone ($\sim 75\%$)
3. Radiopaque
4. Formed in an alkaline urine
5. Etiology
   a. Hypercalciuria
      i. Primary hyerparathyroidism
      ii. Sarcoidosis
      iii. Vitamin D intoxication
      iv. Milk-alkali syndrome
      v. Malignancy
      vi. Idiopathic
   b. Hyperuricosuria (uric acid acts as nidus for calcium stone formation)
   c. Hyperoxaluria
      i. Idiopathic
      ii. Ileal disease, resection or bypass
   d. Renal tubular acidosis

### Uric acid stones

1. Radiolucent
2. Formed in an acid urine
3. Etiology:
   a. Gout
   b. High purine diet
   c. Idiopathic hyperuricemia
   d. Ileostomy, colostomy
   e. Familial

### Cystine stones

1. Radiopaque
2. Etiology: cystinuria only

## RENAL STONES (cont.)

### Struvite stones

1. Magnesium ammonium phosphate
2. Radiopaque
3. May appear as staghorn calculi
4. Formed only in urine of very high pH
5. Etiology: infection with urea-splitting bacteria which generate ammonium from urea (*Klebsiella, Proteus, Pseudomonas, E. coli*)

## ACUTE RENAL FAILURE: KEY FINDINGS OF COMMON CAUSES

| Disorder | Cause | Physical Exam | UA | Other Laboratory Tests | X-ray Ultrasound | Angiography |
|---|---|---|---|---|---|---|
| **Immunologic:** | | | | | | |
| Glomerulo-nephritis | Group A strep (nephritogenic M type) infection | — | + protein + RBCs + RBC casts | Incr. ASO titer Decr. C3 | — | bx. |
| Interstitial nephritis | Drug exposure | Rash | 1+ protein, few cells, casts | Incr. eosinophils | — | bx. |
| Acute tubular necrosis | Radiopaque dye | — | Diverse casts | See following list | — | — |
| SLE | Autoimmune | — | Protein, RBCs, RBC casts | Decr. C3, + ANA | — | — |
| **Obstructive:** | | | | | | |
| **Intrarenal obstruction:** | | | | | | |
| Urate neph-ropathy | Recent chemo-therapy | — | Uric acid crystals | Incr. uric acid in serum and urine | — | — |
| Sulfon-amide crystals | Sulfonamide use | — | Crystals | — | — | — |
| Calcium | Malignancy, endocrine dis-order | Band kerato-pathy | Incr. serum Ca++ generally present | Incr. Ca++ | Nephrocalcinosis | — |

*(continued)*

## ACUTE RENAL FAILURE: KEY FINDINGS OF COMMON CAUSES (cont.)

| Disorder | Cause | Physical Exam | UA | Other Laboratory Tests | X-ray Ultrasound | Angiography |
|---|---|---|---|---|---|---|
| Protein, amyloid, globulins | Multiple myeloma, other hypergammaglobulinemic states | — | Bence-Jones proteins in 40–50% of patients with myeloma | Incr. immunoglobulin in serum | | |
| Extrarenal obstruction: | | | | | | |
| Ureteral | Prior abdominal surgery, trauma | — | — | — | Hydronephrosis | Retrograde dye study |
| Prostatic | Prostatism | Large prostate | — | — | Dilated drainage system | Incr. postvoiding residual |
| Infectious: | | | | | | |
| Acute pyelonephritis | Fever, chills, body pain, dysuria; frequent UTIs | CVA tenderness | WBCs, bacteria | Urine culture positive | — | — |
| Septicemia (incl. bacterial endocarditis) | Primary site of infection | — | Protein RBCs, RBC casts | Blood culture positive | — | — |

*Vascular:*

| | | | | | | |
|---|---|---|---|---|---|---|
| Renal artery obstruction | ASCVD, other embolic events | Incr. BP, bruit | — | — | — | Arteriogram shows lesion; IVP shows delayed filling |
| Acute tubular necrosis | Shock, anaphylaxis | Signs of shock | +protein, muddy brown casts | See following list | — | — |
| Renal vein obstruction | Malignancy or hypercoagulable state | Edema | Incr. protein | — | — | IVP shows defect |
| Prerenal azotemia | Blood loss, dehydration, decr. cardiac output | Signs of hypovolemia or decr. cardiac output | — | See following list | — | — |
| Preeclampsia | Third trimester pregnancy | Incr. edema, BP, proteinuria | — | — | — | — |
| Malignant hypertension | Severe high BP | Incr. BP, retinopathy | — | Proteinuria, sparse casts | — | Biopsy |

*(continued)*

## ACUTE RENAL FAILURE: KEY FINDINGS OF COMMON CAUSES *(cont.)*

| Disorder | Cause | Physical Exam | UA | Other Laboratory Tests | X-ray Ultrasound | Angiography |
|---|---|---|---|---|---|---|
| Hepatorenal syndrome | Hepatic decompensation | Ascites, jaundice, stigma of cirrhosis | — | Picture similar to prerenal azotimia except U(Na⁺) sometimes < 5 mg | — | — |
| Papillary necrosis | SS disease, analgesic abuse | — | — | Urine fails to concentrate to >1.010 | Papillae missing | — |
| Toxic | Exposure to myoglobin, antibiotics, (especially aminoglycosides and cephalosporins), amphotericin B, heavy metals, organic solvents, analgesics (especially phenacetin), heroin, contrast media, and anaesthetic agents (methoxyflurane) | — | — | — | — | — |

## PRERENAL AZOTEMIA VS. ACUTE RENAL FAILURE

Patients with reduced cardiac output, secondary to hypovolemia or cardiac disease, or with the hepatorenal syndrome, may present with a clinical picture very much like acute renal failure: evidence of extracellular fluid depletion and elevated BUN and creatinine levels. It is important to recognize patients with this syndrome of prerenal azotemia, since volume replacement is all the therapy that is required. The following laboratory values can help distinguish between the two conditions. Frequently, the results one obtains may not fall clearly into one or the other category, in which case the $FE_{Na}$ will usually be decisive. Clinically, a volume challenge of several hundred cc's of normal saline may resolve the issue, restoring urine flow in patients with prerenal azotemia.

|  | *Acute Renal Failure* | *Prerenal Azotemia* |
|---|---|---|
| $\dfrac{[\text{Serum BUN}]}{[\text{Serum creatinine}]}$ | <15:1 | >15:1* |
| [Urine Na⁺] | >40 mEq/L | <20 mEq/L |
| Urine osmolality | <350 mOsm/kg | >500 mOsm/kg |
| $\dfrac{[\text{Urine creatinine}]}{[\text{Serum creatinine}]}$ | <20 | >40 |
| Urine specific gravity | 1.010–1.012 | ~1.020 |
| Renal failure index† | >2 | <1 |
| $FE_{Na}$‡ | >2 | <1 |

*An elevated BUN out of proportion to the creatinine can also be seen with GI bleeding, steroid therapy, tetracycline therapy, and hyperalimentation.

†The renal failure index is calculated in this way:

$$\frac{[\text{Urine Na}]}{[\text{Urine creatinine}]/[\text{Plasma creatinine}]}$$

‡The $FE_{Na}$, or fractional excretion of filtered sodium, is calculated in this way:

$$\frac{[\text{Urine Na}]/[\text{Plasma Na}]}{[\text{Urine creatinine}]/[\text{Plasma creatinine}]}$$

## THE UREMIC SYNDROME: MANIFESTATIONS

1. Cutaneous
   a. Pruritis
   b. Hyperpigmentation
   c. Uremic frost
2. Neurologic
   a. Peripheral: sensory polyneuropathy, distal motor dysfunction
   b. Central: insomnia, short attention span, clonus, asterixis, encephalopathy, seizures, coma
3. Cardiac
   a. Accelerated atherosclerosis
   b. Hypertension
   c. Arrhythmias
   d. Cardiomyopathy
   e. Congestive heart failure
   f. Pericarditis
   g. Cardiac tamponade
4. Pulmonary
   a. Edema
   b. Interstitial fibrosis
   c. Pleural effusions
5. Hematologic
   a. Anemia
   b. Mild hemolysis
   c. Platelet dysfunction (increased bleeding time often without thrombocytopenia)
   d. Leukopenia
   e. Impaired neutrophil function
6. Gastrointestinal
   a. Nausea, vomiting
   b. Anorexia
   c. Mouth ulcers
   d. Parotitis
   e. Mild GI bleeding

7. Metabolic
   a. Weight loss
   b. Glucose intolerance
   c. Elevated serum triglycerides
   d. Metabolic acidosis
   e. Hyperkalemia
   f. Hyponatremia
   g. Hypermagnesemia
7. Calcium, phosphorus, and bone
   a. Hyperphosphatemia
   b. Hypocalcemia
   c. Vitamin D deficiency
   d. Secondary hyperparathyroidism
   e. Metastatic calcification
   f. Osteitis fibrosa captica
8. Increased susceptibility to infection
9. Sexual dysfunction

## DETERMINING THE PRIMARY SITE OF
## INTRINSIC RENAL DISEASE

| | Glomerular Disease (e.g., chronic glomerulonephritis, nephrotic syndrome) | Interstitial Disease (e.g., pyelonephritis, acute interstitial nephritis) | Tubular Disease (e.g., acute tubular necrosis) |
|---|---|---|---|
| Proteinuria | Heavy | Light | Light |
| Epithelial cells, RBC's and WBC's | + | + | + |
| Casts: | | | |
|   Hyaline | + | + | + |
|   RBC | + | Unusual | Unusual |
|   WBC | Variable | + | Unusual |
|   Epithelial cell | Variable | Unusual | + |
|   Granular | Variable | Variable | + |
|   Waxy | + | Unusual | Unusual |
| Urine culture | − | +/− | − |
| Hypertension | Common | Variable | Variable |
| Anemia | + when uremic | + | Unusual |
| Compromise of tubular functions (fluid and electrolyte imbalances, impaired concentrating ability) | Unusual until late in course | + | + |

## ACUTE VS. CHRONIC RENAL FAILURE

**Establishing the Duration of Renal Deterioration in a Patient with No History of Preexisting Renal Disease**

1. History is suggestive. How long has patient been symptomatic? Has there been any acute insult, especially one associated with hypovolemia or hypotension?
2. A profusion of uremic symptoms generally signifies chronic renal disease, but not always. Two manifestations of the uremic syndrome, however, are present only in chronic disease: osteitis fibrosa (documented by bone x-ray) and peripheral neuropathy.
3. The finding of small kidneys on abdominal x-ray or sonography generally indicates chronic renal failure. However, some cases of chronic disease are associated with normal-sized kidneys: diabetic nephropathy, amyloidosis, rapidly progressive glomerulonephritis, and even some cases of chronic glomerulonephritis.
4. Renal biopsy is a definitive procedure, establishing the precise etiology in the vast majority of patients.

## REMEDIABLE CAUSES OF CHRONIC RENAL FAILURE

1. Obstruction (usually stones)
2. Infection (usually pyelonephritis)
3. Systemic diseases
    a. SLE
    b. Gout
    c. Hypertension
    d. Diabetes
    e. Wegener's granulomatosis
4. Nephrotoxic drugs
    a. Phenacetin
    b. Antibiotics
    c. Amphotericin B
    d. Heroin
    e. Methoxyflurane
5. Heavy metals
6. Metabolic disorders
    a. Hypercalcemia
    b. Hyperuricemia

## EFFECTIVENESS AND COMPLICATIONS
## OF HEMODIALYSIS

1. Uremic manifestations that usually respond favorably
   a. CNS abnormalities
   b. Gastrointestinal involvement
   c. Bleeding
   d. Weight loss
   e. Fluid and electrolyte disorders
   f. Glucose intolerance
2. Uremic manifestations that usually persist
   a. Anemia
   b. Hypertension
   c. Pericarditis
   d. Cardiovascular disease (especially atherosclerosis)
   e. Bone disease
   f. Sexual dysfunction
   g. Increased susceptibility to infection
   h. Pruritis
   i. Peripherial neuropathy (progession may be halted, but the neural involvement is rarely reversed)
3. Complications
   a. Difficulty in creating and maintaining vascular access
   b. Shunt infection
   c. Infectious hepatitis
   d. Hypotension
   e. Insomnia
   f. Bleeding (usually related to anticoagulation, which is frequently given to maintain the patency of the vascular access site)
   g. Dialysis disequilibrium, a syndrome that may include headache, nausea, vomiting, fatigue, weakness, muscle cramps (especially in the legs), visual blurring, anxiety and paresthesias; it may progress to seizures and psychosis
   h. Dialysis dementia may occur after several years of dialysis, and may include dementia, seizures, and psychosis
   i. Depression (the suicide rate of patients on chronic dialysis is significantly greater than the normal population)

## EFFECTIVENESS AND COMPLICATIONS
## OF HEMODIALYSIS *(cont.)*

4. Cause of death in patients on chronic hemodialysis

| Cause | Percent |
|---|---|
| a. Cardiovascular (mostly CVA and MI) | 50% |
| b. Sepsis | 25% |
| c. Suicide | 5–10% |
| d. Other | 15–20% |

## WHEN TO INSTITUTE HEMODIALYSIS

### Absolute Indications

1. Severe oliguria or anuria
2. Malignant hypertension unresponsive to therapy
3. Encephalopathy or coma
4. Hyperkalemia with cardiographic changes
5. Coagulopathy
6. Severe metabolic acidosis
7. Pericarditis
8. Severe peripheral motor neuropathy
9. Volume overload resistant to conservative measures

### Preferred

When possible, dialysis should be instituted before the onset of any of the absolute indications above. Hemodialysis is frequently begun in patients with continued progression of uremic manifestations (especially those manifestations that respond favorably to dialysis, see list on page 207) and when conservative therapy is inadequate to maintain an acceptable quality of life.

# Section

# 8

# Gastroenterology

## COMMON CAUSES OF ABDOMINAL PAIN: CHARACTERISTIC FEATURES

### Peptic Ulcer Disease

1. Location: midepigastric.
2. Description: episodic, burning, gnawing pain, recurring over several weeks; food usually provides relief of duodenal ulcer pain, but may worsen gastric ulcer pain.
3. Findings: epigastric tenderness.
4. An upper GI barium study or endoscopy is the diagnostic test of choice.
5. Perforation presents with sudden sharp abdominal pain, typically radiating to the right shoulder. On chest x-ray, free air can often be seen under the diaphragm. Signs of peritonitis and shock may quickly dominate the clinical picture. The serum amylase may be elevated in posterior perforations.
6. Other significant complications of peptic ulcer disease include bleeding, recurring pain, and gastric outlet obstruction.

### Pancreatitis

1. Location: epigastric, often radiating to the back.
2. Description: severe pain, with nausea and vomiting, sometimes eased by bending forward.
3. Findings: in uncomplicated pancreatitis—gastric tenderness, hypoactive bowel sounds; with peritonitis—fever, hypotension, tachycardia, pallor and rebound tenderness. An abdominal mass may be felt with pseudocyst formation. Rarely, signs of respiratory distress may be noted.
4. History of alcoholism or biliary tract disease is common.
5. Elevated serum amylase and urinary amylase clearance; decreased serum calcium is an ominous sign.
6. X-ray may reveal pancreatic calcification, a widened duodenal sweep or a sentinel loop.
7. Ultrasound may reveal a pancreatic mass.

### Cholecystitis

1. Location: right upper quadrant, may radiate to right scapula.
2. Description: severe and steady pain (despite the term "biliary colic") usually accompanied by nausea and vomiting.

3. Findings: fever, hypoactive bowel sounds, right upper quadrant tenderness; an enlarged gallbladder may be palpable; positive Murphy's sign (pain upon palpation below the right costal margin causes inspiratory arrest).
4. Jaundice with dark urine and light stools may accompany obstruction of the common duct.
5. Serum bilirubin and alkaline phosphatase are elevated.
6. X-ray and ultrasound may reveal stones; a Hida scan can be very useful and is considered by many the diagnostic test of choice.

## Appendicitis

1. Location: pain typically begins in the epigastrium and later localizes to the right lower quadrant.
2. Description: gradual in onset with nausea, vomiting, anorexia.
3. Findings: low grade fever, right lower quadrant rebound tenderness, and tenderness on rectal exam; signs of peritonitis develop with perforation.
4. Typical progression of symptoms:
   a. Pain, often predominantly midepigastric
   b. Nausea and vomiting
   c. Tenderness over appendix
   d. Fever and leukocytosis
5. X-ray may reveal localized ileus or increased soft tissue density obscuring the psoas margin.

## Diverticulitis

1. Location: left lower quadrant, although often initially hypogastric.
2. Description: like "left-sided appendicitis" with a change in bowel habits and anorexia (the latter is less prominent than in appendicitis).
3. Findings: quiet bowel sounds, left lower quadrant tenderness, left-sided fullness or mass may be palpated, localized peritonitis, evidence of obstruction may be present (see below).
4. Barium enema reveals diverticulae.

## COMMON CAUSES OF ABDOMINAL PAIN: CHARACTERISTIC FEATURES *(cont.)*

### Bowel obstruction

1. Location: depends on site of obstruction
2. Description: crampy pain with nausea, vomiting, constipation
3. Findings: fever is absent, bowel sounds are high-pitched and often hyperactive, there is minimal tenderness
4. X-ray may reveal dilatation of the bowel with air-fluid levels

### Inflammatory Bowel Disease

1. Location: periumbilical or lower abdominal
2. Description: crampy pain with anorexia, weight loss, vomiting, a change in bowel habits and sometimes bloody diarrhea (the last only in ulcerative colitis)
3. Findings: tenderness over the site of involvement, extra-articular manifestations are common (arthritis and skin involvement, especially)
4. X-ray:
   a. Ulcerative colitis—ulcerations, strictures, polyps, absence of haustral markings
   b. Regional enteritis—intestinal strictures, narrowings, and fistulae with stretches of normal bowel between; cobblestone bowel; string sign

### Bowel infarction

1. Location: periumbilical, poorly localized.
2. Description: crampy pain that gradually worsens and then becomes constant.
3. Findings: distention and evidence of obstruction may be present, evidence of sepsis, shock, or peritonitis may dominate the clinical picture; blood eventually can be detected in the stool and/or vomitus.
4. Many patients have a history of vascular disease.
5. X-ray reveals ileus and thickening of the bowel wall.
6. Lab studies may reveal an elevated WBC, amylase, and frequently, lactate with an elevated anion gap.

## CAUSES OF GASTROINTESTINAL BLEEDING

1. Upper GI
   a. Esophageal varices
   b. Esophagitis
   c. Mallory-Weiss tear
   d. Esophageal carcinoma
   e. Gastric ulcer
   f. Gastritis
   g. Gastric carcinoma
   h. Duodenal ulcer
2. Lower GI
   a. Inflammatory bowel disease
   b. Tumors
   c. Meckel's diverticulum
   d. Diverticulitis
   e. Bowel infarction
   f. Polyps
   g. Enterocolitis
   h. Angiodysplasia
   i. Hemorrhoids

Note: Any pathologic site is more likely to bleed when a concomitant coagulation disorder exists.

## ACUTE GI BLEED: WORKUP

1. Assess extent of blood lost:
   a. Pressure drop of 10 mm Hg and pulse augmentation of 20 beats/minute when patient is moved from supine to sitting or standing position generally occur with loss of 20% blood volume.
   b. Shock (hypotension and tachycardia in supine position) generally signifies loss of 40–50% blood volume.
2. Initial steps:
   a. Insert at least two 14–18 guage IV lines. Isotonic saline should be given until transfusion can begin.
   b. Obtain blood studies:
      i. Type and crossmatch
      ii. Serum electrolytes
      iii. Clotting parameters (needed for fresh frozen plasma, vitamin K, or platelets)
      iv. Creatinine
      v. Liver function tests
      vi. Hematocrit (cannot be used to assess extent of blood lost)
   c. Establish a CVP line to assess changes in blood volume during therapy, if patient has severe underlying cardiac disease
   d. Other studies:
      i. Urine output
      ii. ECG, especially in elderly patients
3. Transfusion with whole blood [O⁻ if necessary] or packed RBCs and crystalloid in patients with clinical evidence of hypovolemia is started as soon as possible. Blood may need to be given at a rate of 1 unit every 20–30 minutes to achieve and maintain an adequate hematocrit ($>30\%$) and CVP ($>8$ cm $H_2O$). One unit of cells should raise the hematocrit 3–4% after equilibration of approximately 8 hours.
4. Localize the bleeding (upper or lower)
   a. Hematemesis usually signifies bleeding proximal to the jejunum; melena results from contact of blood with gastric secretions, and therefore suggests upper GI bleeding, but may result from small bowel bleeding if transit time is slow.

    b. Rectal exam and stool guaiac

    c. Pass a nasogastric tube and infuse a small volume of saline. Aspirate contents:

       i. Bright red blood signifies active upper GI bleeding, and an iced saline lavage can be started.

      ii. Coffee grounds material signifies a recent bleed that has stopped.

     iii. Absence of blood in the aspirate can be due to an intermittent bleed, a lower GI bleed, incorrect tube placement, or can occur with duodenal bleeding in the presence of a deformed pylorus.

    d. A history of previous episodes of localized GI bleeding is helpful, but many patients (>40% of alcoholics) rebleed from a second site.

5. Determine the specific site of bleeding.

    a. If upper GI:

       i. Contrast studies (simplest to perform, but give the smallest diagnostic yield).

      ii. Endoscopy if bleeding can be lavaged to pink or clear.

     iii. Arteriography if endoscopy is unsuccessful; if a lesion is visualized, a select vasopression infusion can be tried).

    b. If lower GI:

       i. Proctosigmoidoscopy

      ii. Colonoscopy

     iii. Angiography (selective vasopression can then be tried)

     iv. Contrast studies

6. In patients with bleeding varices, selective vasopression infusions may halt the bleeding. If this fails, a Sengstaken-Blakemore tube can be tried. Sclerosis and surgery are other options.

## TREATMENT OF PEPTIC ULCER DISEASE

### Principal Agents

The principal agents for the medical management of peptic ulcer disease are antacids and cimetidine.

1. Absorbable antacids (not recommended for chronic use)
   a. Sodium bicarbonate—side effects are alkalosis, sodium and fluid retention.
   b. Calcium bicarbonate—side effects are acid rebound, constipation, hypercalcemia, renal damage, milk-alkali syndrome (a syndrome of hypercalcemia and alkalosis, which can lead to renal insufficiency; it is usually associated with the ingestion of large quantities of milk).
2. Nonabsorbable antacids
   a. Aluminum compounds (Amphojel, Basaljel, Phosphajel)—side effects are constipation, phosphate depletion, binding of certain drugs (e.g., tetracycline), and accelerating the absorption of others (e.g., diazepam).
   b. Magnesium compounds (Milk of Magnesia)—side effects are diarrhea, hypermagnesemia in patients with renal failure.
   c. Mixtures of aluminum hydroxide and magnesium hydroxide (Mylanta, Gelusil, Maalox, Maalox Plus, Riopan)—These mixtures were designed to balance the laxative and constipating effects of magnesium and aluminum compounds, respectively. Mylanta, Gelusil and Maalox Plus also contain simethicone, a mixture touted as effective in reducing gas (defoaming) and thereby able to reduce the risk of gastroesophageal reflux.
3. Cimetidine: a blocker of the histamine $H_2$ receptor. Side effects: endocrine dysfunction in males has been reported (impotence, gynecomastia), confusion and disorientation in the elderly.

## Principles of Therapy

1. The most common mistake in treating peptic ulcer disease is to give too little antacid too infrequently. A gastric pH of 5 is necessary to abolish pepsin action.
2. Acute ulcer pain can be treated with frequent small feedings, reduced activity and psychological stress, and hourly antacids.
3. After the acute attack has subsided, antacids can be given 1 and 3 hours after every meal and before bed time.
4. Chronic treatment may include frequent small feedings and antacids given 1 hour every meal and before bed time.
5. Cimetidine can be given every 6 hours, usually with meals and at bedtime. It has been shown to be effective in reducing acid secretion and hastening healing and reducing pain in duodenal ulcers.

## CAUSES OF AN ENLARGED LIVER

1. Inflammation
   a. Infectious hepatitis
   b. Drug-related (toxic) hepatitis
   c. Alcoholic hepatitis
2. Cirrhosis
   a. Alcoholic
   b. Nonalcoholic (e.g., primary biliary cirrhosis, Wilson's disease)
3. Infiltrative disease
   a. Primary and metastatic tumors
   b. Lymphoma and leukemia
   c. Extramedullary hematopoiesis
   d. Amyloidosis
   e. Hemachromatosis
   f. Glycogen storage diseases
4. Biliary tract obstruction
   a. Gallstones
   b. Pancreatic cancer
   c. Tumor of the common bile duct or ampulla of Vater
5. Venous congestion
   a. Congestive heart failure
   b. Constrictive pericarditis

With *acute* enlargement, the liver is tender, soft and smooth. Ascites is rare. The serum albumin is usually normal, but the SGOT is elevated, often to very high levels.

With *chronic* enlargement, the liver is nontender, firm, and finely nodular (large nodules or irregular masses imply malignancy). Ascites is common. The serum albumin is often decreased, and the SGOT is normal or elevated, although never to the dramatic levels frequently seen in acute inflammation.

## JAUNDICE

Jaundice develops when the serum bilirubin exceeds 2–3 mg/dL. The skin, sclerae, and mucous membranes acquire a yellowish tint, the urine becomes dark, and the stool may become light.

## Pathway of Bilirubin Metabolism

1. Within the reticuloendothelial system, dying red blood cells release free hemoglobin.
2. The heme moiety is converted to biliverdin and then to bilirubin, which is bound tightly to serum albumin for transport. Bilirubin bound to albumin cannot be excreted in the urine.
3. Bilirubin enters the liver where it is separated from albumin and conjugated to glucuronic acid. If conjugated ("direct") bilirubin is regurgitated into the circulation, it binds poorly to albumin and can appear in the urine.
4. Conjugated bilirubin is excreted into the bile and then into the intestine.
5. Some of this excreted bilirubin appears in the stool; the remainder is converted to urobilinogen. Urobilinogen can be resorbed in the distal ileum and reexcreted in bile or urine.

## Differential Diagnosis of Jaundice

A precise etiologic diagnosis is essential for separating medically treatable causes of jaundice from those requiring surgery.

| Etiology | Initial Mode of Therapy | Key Diagnostic Points |
|---|---|---|
| *Unconjugated hyperbilirubinemia* | | |
| Benign, inherited disorders Gilbert's syndrome | None | No evidence of illness, normal liver function tests, positive family history |
| Severe hemolysis Immunologic, mechanical (value prosthesis), sickle cell anemia, G-6-PD deficiency, hereditary spherocytosis | Medical | No bilirubinuria, evidence of anemia |

## JAUNDICE *(cont.)*

| Etiology | Initial Mode of Therapy | Key Diagnostic Points |
|---|---|---|
| *Unconjugated hyperbilirubinemia* | | |
| Benign, inherited disorders Dubin-Johnson syndrome | None | Bilirubinuria, no evidence of illness, jaundice often first appears during pregnancy, characteristic liver biopsy |
| Liver disease Viral and toxic hepatitis, cirrhosis, neoplasia (primary and metastatic), and infiltrative disease (e.g., amyloidosis) | Medical | Bilirubinuria, prolonged prothrombin time not corrected with vitamin K, SGOT may be very high in acute hepatitis |
| Extrahepatic obstruction Gallbladder disease, tumor obstructing the common bite duct, carcinoma of the ampulla of Vater, pancreatic cancer | Surgical | Bilirubinuria, prolonged prothrombin time is corrected with vitamin K, SGOT rarely exceeds 300 IU, pruritis is common |

## SITES OF OBSTRUCTION IN
## PORTAL HYPERTENSION

| Disease | Frequency | Location of obstruction |
|---|---|---|
| Extrahepatic portal vein occlusion | Rare | Portal vein |
| Schistosomiasis | Common in endemic areas | Tiny portal veins |
| Metastatic nodules | Common | Tiny portal veins |
| Extramedullary hematopoeisis | Common | Tiny portal veins |
| Lipid or amyloid accumulation | Common | Portal sinusoids |
| Hypertrophic endoplasmic reticulum secondary to increased flow or splenomegaly | Rare | Portal sinusoids |
| Cirrhosis (alcoholic or postnecrotic) | Common | Portal sinusoids |
| Budd-Chiari syndrome | Rare | Hepatic veins |
| Venocclusive disease | Rare | Hepatic veins |
| Vena caval obstruction | Uncommon | Vena cava and hepatic veins |
| Constrictive pericarditis or right-sided congestive heart failure | Common | Right atrium |

## FEATURES OF VIRAL HEPATITIS

| Characteristic | Hepatitis A ("infectious") | Hepatitis B ("serum") | Non-A, Non-B Hepatitis |
|---|---|---|---|
| Spread | Fecal-oral, raw shellfish. | Blood, blood products, saliva, semen | Blood, blood products (80–90% of posttransfusion hepatitis cases) |
| Incubation period | 15–50 days (average 28 ±7) | 45–80 days (average 75 ±25) | 35–70 days |
| Prodrome (fever, weight loss, rash, headache, nausea, vomiting, abdominal pain, myalgias, arthralgias, lassitude, dark urine, light stools | Abrupt, less than 5 days | Less than 30 days; in 10–20% includes arthralgias, urticaria, angioedema | Gradual |
| Viremia | Transient, over by onset of jaundice | Persistent | — |
| Chronic carriers | No | 10% | — |
| Duration of elevated transaminases | 1–3 weeks | 1–6 months | — |

| | | | |
|---|---|---|---|
| Mortality | Very rare, 0–0.2% | Rarely (0.3–15%), patients may develop acute fulminant hepatitis, which frequently culminates in death | Rare, probably similar to hepatitis A |
| Progression to chronic active hepatitis | No | Approximately 10% | 10–40%(?) |
| Protection with gamma globulin | Ordinary gamma globulin (0.02 mL/kg) causes an 8-fold decreased incidence in populations at risk | Hyperimmune gamma globulin (5 ml, repeat at 1 month) causes a 3–10-fold decreased incidence in populations at risk | Ordinary gamma globulin slightly decreases incidences in populations at risk |
| Protection with vaccine | None | 95% effective | None |

# VIRAL HEPATITIS: INTERPRETING TEST RESULTS

| HB$_s$Ag | Anti-HB$_s$ | Anti-HB$_c$ | HB$_e$AG | Anti-HB$_e$ | HAVAB | | Interpretation |
| | | | | | IgM | IgG | |
|---|---|---|---|---|---|---|---|
| Negative | Negative | Negative | — | — | — | — | Probably not HBV* |
| — | — | — | — | — | Negative | Negative | Probably not HAV* |
| Positive | Negative | Negative | — | — | — | — | Early HBV |
| Positive | Negative | Positive | — | — | — | — | HBV infection acute or chronic; chronic carrier state |
| Positive | — | — | Positive | Negative | — | — | Patient is probably infectious |
| Positive | — | — | Negative | Positive | — | — | Patient is probably not infectious |
| Negative | Negative | Positive | — | — | — | — | Persistent HBV or early convalescence |
| Negative | Positive | Positive | — | — | — | — | Recovery from HBV, immunity developing 2–4 months after illness |
| Negative | Positive | Negative | — | — | — | — | Immune to HBV (5–15% of population |
| — | — | — | — | — | Positive | Negative | Acute HAV |
| — | — | — | — | — | Negative | Positive | Immune to HAV (30–45% of U.S.) |

## Suggested Evaluation of Viral Hepatitis

1. To diagnose HBV (dialysis patients, drug addicts, persons with sexual contact with HB$_s$AG positive persons): HB$_s$AG and HB$_c$Ab.

2. To diagnose HAV (food associated epidemics, sporadic case with no history of contact with HB$_s$Ag person or parenteral drug use): HAVAb IgM and IgG.

3. To decide about use of HB immune globulin (HBIG) (needle sticks, infants of HB$_s$Ag mothers, sexual contacts with HB$_s$Ag-positive persons): "Donor"—HB$_e$AG; "Recipient"—HB$_s$AG (if +, then HBIG not needed).

4. For evaluation of carrier infectivity: HB$_e$Ag and HB$_e$Ab.

*Persons with signs and symptoms of hepatitis with persisting negative tests for one month are assumed to have non-A, non-B hepatitis.

## DIFFERENTIATING CHRONIC ACTIVE FROM CHRONIC PERSISTENT HEPATITIS

1. Chronic active hepatitis
   a. Clinical manifestations
      i. Onset: usually insidious over several weeks to months although in one third of patients it is only 1–2 weeks, resembling acute viral hepatitis.
      ii. Description: marked constitutional symptoms (fatigue, malaise, anorexia), abdominal pain, hepatosplenomegaly, low grade fever; jaundice in 80% of patients; extrahepatic involvement (arthralgias, colitis, pleuritis, pericarditis, sicca syndrome, skin lesions) is common.
   b. Laboratory
      i. SGOT, SGPT: usually > 100 IU, often > 400 IU.
      ii. Bilirubin: often > 3 mg/100 mL.
      iii. Prothrombin time: prolonged.
      iv. Albumin: often decreased.
      v. Serum immunoglobulins: usually increased.
      vi. Antinuclear antibodies: positive in up to 50% of patients.
      vii. Smooth muscle antibodies: positive in up to 80% of patients.
      viii. $HB_sAg$: positive in 10–30% of patients.
   c. Liver biobsy: lobular architecture is severely altered with fibrosis, inflammation extending beyond the portal areas, piecemeal necrosis and evidence of hepatic regeneration.
   d. Course: variable and progressive, leading to cirrhosis and liver failure; 5-year survival without treatment is less than 50%.
2. Chronic persistent hepatitis
   a. Clinical manifestations
      i. Onset: typically over 1–2 weeks, resembling acute vital hepatitis.
      ii. Description: mild constitutional symptoms, abdominal pain, hepatosplenomegaly, low-grade fever; jaundice and extrahepatic involvement are rare.

b. Laboratory
   i. SGOT, SGPT: 40–200 IU (may abruptly rise higher, then recede).
   ii. Bilirubin: < 3 mg/100 mL.
   iii. Prothrombin time: usually normal.
   iv. Albumin: usually normal.
   v. Serum immunoglobulins: normal or slightly elevated.
   vi. Antinuclear antibodies: rarely positive.
   vii. Smooth muscle antibodies: rarely positive.
   viii. $HB_S Ag$: positive in 10–30% of patients.
c. Liver biopsy: lobular architecture is maintained, mild periportal inflammation and little fibrosis.
d. Course: not progressive with no increased mortality; therapy is not required.

## COMMON DRUGS THAT CAN DAMAGE THE LIVER

1. Anesthetics: halothane, nitrous oxide, methoxyflurane, chloroform
2. Antibacterial: sulfonamides, tetracycline, erythromycin, penicillins
3. Antituberculosis: isoniazid, rifampicin, PAS
4. Neuro- and psychopharmacologic: chlorpromazine, phenytoin, amitryptiline, meperidine, diazepam
5. Oral contraceptives
6. Analgesics: acetaminophen, phenylbutazone, salicylates
7. Methyldopa
8. Toxins: mushrooms (*Amanita phalloides*), carbon tetrachloride, vinyl chloride

## ASCITES

### Diagnostic Paracentesis

In all patients with undiagnosed ascites, the following tests should be performed on a sample of the aspirated fluid (100 ml is usually sufficient):

1. Note gross appearance. Milky fluid implies lymphatic obstruction (chylous ascites), thick turbid fluid is seen with inflammation, clear fluid implies cirrhosis or obstruction, and bloody fluid may be seen with malignancies.
2. Protein. A protein concentration above 2.5–3.0 gm/dL is indicative of an exudative process (infection or malignancy), whereas a protein concentration below 2.5 gm/dL indicates a transudative disorder (cirrhosis or nephrosis).
3. Glucose. Levels markedly below the serum level can be seen with infection or malignancy.
4. Amylase. Elevated levels (around 500 units) imply pancreatic ascites, but may also be seen with intestinal and ovarian disease.
5. White blood count. Only rarely helpful. An elevated absolute white count or a high percentage of PMNs may indicate peritonitis.
6. Cytology. Malignant cells must be searched for.
7. Gram stain, acid-fast stain, and bacterial cultures. Infection must be considered a possibility in all patients.

### Causes

1. Transudative ascites
   a. Hepatic lesions
      i. Cirrhosis
      ii. Malignancies (these more commonly produce exudates)
      iii. Granulomatous diseases
   b. Other lesions
      i. Congestive heart failure
      ii. Constrictive pericarditis
      iii. Venous blockage (e.g., Budd-Chiari syndrome)
      iv. Hypoalbuminemia (e.g., nephrotic syndrome or protein losing gastroenteropathy)
      v. Gynecologic disease (e.g., Meig's syndrome or struma ovarii)

## ASCITES *(cont.)*

2. Exudative ascites
   a. Inflammation (peritonitis)
      i. Rupture of an abdominal organ (as may occur in peptic ulcer disease, appendicitis, diverticulitis, etc.)
      ii. Spontaneous bacterial peritonitis
      iii. Tuberculosis
      iv. Pancreatitis
      v. Bile peritonitis
      vi. Rarely, fungal or parasitic infection
   b. Malignancy
      i. Hepatoma
      ii. Metastasis to the liver or peritoneum
      iii. Leukemia, lymphoma
   c. Myxedema
3. Chylous ascites
   a. Mediastinal malignancy
   b. Trauma to the thoracic duct
   c. Filariasis
   d. Rarely, tuberculosis
4. Mucinous ascites (*Pseudomyxoma peritonei*): mucinous tumors, usually of the ovary or appendix

## HEPATIC ENCEPHALOPATHY

1. Manifestations
   a. Gradually deteriorating mental function marked by lethargy, confusion, irritability, and impaired judgment.
   b. Asterixis (also seen in uremia and $CO_2$ narcosis)
   c. Myoclonus
   d. Hyperventilation (producing a respiratory alkalosis)
   e. Coma
2. Common precipitating factors in patients with severe liver disease
   a. Excess nitrogen load
      i. Excess protein in diet
      ii. Gastrointestinal bleeding
      iii. Uremia
      iv. Constipation
      v. Infection
   b. Drugs: sedatives, tranquilizers, narcotics, diuretics
   c. Hypokalemia and/or hypovolemia: often related to diuretic use
3. Principles of management
   a. Identify and treat any precipitating factors.
   b. Restrict protein.
   c. Cleanse bowel with enemas or laxatives.
   d. Then, administer neomycin or lactulose. Neomycin reduces the nitrogen load, presumably by sterilizing the bowel. Side effects result from systemic absorption of a small percent of the drug, and include nephrotoxicity and ototoxicity. Lactulose acts as a cathartic and also traps ammonia in the gut by lowering the intestinal pH. It is safer than neomycin and equally as effective.

## PATHOPHYSIOLOGY OF SIGNS AND SYMPTOMS IN PANCREATITIS

| *Clinical feature* | *Pathophysiology* |
|---|---|
| Abdominal pain, fever, ascites | Release and activation of proteases; phospholipases destroy pancreatic tissue and cause retroperitoneal inflammation with fluid accumulation; fluid contains amylase, polymorpho-nuclear cells and red blood cells. |
| Mild jaundice, elevated bilirubin, or alkaline phosphatase | Edema compressing common bile duct; no stone necessary. |
| Tachypnea or pleuritic chest pain | Pleural effusion or pleuritis; impending respiratory distress. |
| Shock | Retroperitoneal loss of protein-rich fluid. Kallikrein activation causes bradykinin production leading to altered capillary permeability and vasodilation, which in turn cause hypotension, decreased urinary output, and, sometimes, acute tubular necrosis. |
| Altered coagulation | Increased fibrinolysis; trypsin converts plasminogen to plasmin, which is fibrinolytic. Trypsin itself digests thrombin. |
| Altered coagulation | Trypsin can convert prothrombin to thrombin. Vessel necrosis causes thrombosis. |
| Fat necrosis (Weber-Christian syndrome) | Local and distal effects of lipase and phospholipase on fat creates $Ca^{++}$ and $Mg^{++}$ soaps. |
| Hypocalcemia and tetany | (?) Increased glucagon secondary to pancreatic necrosis causes increased calcitonin and decreased mobilization of bone calcium. May impede normal restoration of $Ca^{++}$ by PTH. |
| Hyperglycemia (transient) | Decreased production and release of insulin due to pancreatic necrosis; also, adrenal response to stress. |

| | |
|---|---|
| Respiratory distress syndrome | (?) Destruction of lung tissue. (?) Surfactant breakdown by released phospholipases. |
| Hyperlipemia | Decreased clearance of lipoproteins. Mechanism uncertain. In types I and V hyperlipemia, pancreatitis is a common occurrence. |
| Methemalbuminemia | With hemorrhagic necrosis, hemoglobin is digested by proteolytic agents to form ferriheme, which binds to albumin. This finding helps to distinguish hemorrhagic from edematous pancreatitis. |

## AMYLASE

### Hyperamylasemia: Common Causes

Pancreatitis
Pancreatic carcinoma
Parotitis
Ruptured ectopic pregnancy
Intestinal obstruction, infarction, or perforation
Biliary disease
Peptic ulcer disease
Renal insufficiency
Macroamylasemia

### Making the Diagnosis: Calculating the Amylase/Creatinine Clearance Ratio

The above list shows that many causes of abdominal discomfort other than pancreatitis can cause an elevated serum amylase. Only in pancreatitis, however, is the renal resorption of amylase decreased, thus leading to especially high concentrations of urinary amylase. This enhanced amylase clearance is reflected in an increased amylase/creatinine clearance ration calculated by using the formula:

$$\frac{\text{Amylase clearance}}{\text{Creatinine clearance}} = \frac{\text{(Urine amylase)}}{\text{(Serum amylase)}} \times \frac{\text{(Serum creatinine)}}{\text{(Urine creatinine)}}$$

A ratio of greater than 5% is considered diagnostic of pancreatitis. The creatinine clearance is included as a correction factor to eliminate cases where renal failure is responsible for hyperamylasemia.

## DIFFERENTIAL DIAGNOSIS OF ACUTE PANCREATITIS

| Etiology | History | Distinguishing Physical Findings | Lab Findings |
|---|---|---|---|
| Acute pancreatitis | Sudden onset; history of gallstones, EtOH, ulcers, surgery, trauma, hyperlipidemia, thiazides | Abdominal findings moderate compared to pain; tenderness in lower epigastric area; shock, cyanosis, restlessness | Increased amylase in serum and urine; paracentesis reveals amylase, fat necrosis, and, sometimes, blood; chest x-ray may show fluid at left base |
| Perforated viscus, especially duodenal ulcer | History of ulcer | Boardlike spasm and epigastric tenderness | Free air under diaphragm |
| Mesenteric vascular occlusion | Elderly patient; history of recent surgery or artherosclerotic coronary vascular disease; gradual onset | Heme-positive stool | WBC>20,000; ?? bloody stool; positive angiogram |
| Acute intestinal obstruction | Intermittent, colicky pain; history of surgery or tumor | Distention, borborygmi; shock is rare | X-ray shows mechanical obstruction |

*(continued)*

237

## DIFFERENTIAL DIAGNOSIS OF ACUTE PANCREATITIS (cont.)

| Etiology | History | Distinguishing Physical Findings | Lab Findings |
|----------|---------|----------------------------------|--------------|
| Biliary disease | Pain is right sided; gradual onset, less prostrating than pancreatitis | Murphy's sign | Ultrasound, intravenous cholecystography or trans-hepatic cholangiogram shows abnormal gall bladder with or without stones |
| Dissecting aneurysm | Sharp pain, frequently felt in chest and abdomen; history of artherosclerotic coronary vascular disease | Diminished femoral pulses; shock, restlessness | Frequently, hematuria |

## PRINCIPLES OF THERAPY IN ACUTE PANCREATITIS

| *Therapeutic intervention* | *Purpose* |
| --- | --- |
| Nasogastric suction, prohibiting all oral intake, antacid therapy | Decrease both gastrin and acid stimulation of pancreatic secretion |
| Colloid, saline infusions | Treat hypotension |
| ?? Parasympathetic agents | Decrease gastric and pancreatic secretion |
| Calcium gluconate | Treat hypocalcemia |
| Analgesics, frequently narcotic | Treat pain |

## PROGNOSIS IN ACUTE PANCREATITIS*

### Early Objective Signs Used To Classify the Severity of Pancreatitis

At admission or diagnosis:

Age over 55
White blood cell count over 16,000/m$^3$
Blood glucose over 200 mg/100 mL
Serum lactic dehydrogenase over 350 IU/L
Serum glutamic oxaloacetic transaminase over 250 Sigma Frankel
Units/100 mL

During initial 48 hours:

Hematocrit falls more than 10 percentage points
Blood urea nitrogen rises more than 5 mg/100 mL
Serum calcium level below 8 mg/100 mL
Arterial PO$_2$ below 60 mm Hg
Base deficit greater than 4 mEq/L
Estimated fluid sequestration more than 6,000 mL

Patients with <3 signs have a   1% mortality
              3–4 signs        15% mortality
              5–6 signs        40% mortality
              7–8 signs        nearly 100% mortality

*From Ranson GHC, Spencer FC: Am Surg 187:565, 1978.

## ACUTE DIARRHEA: COMMON CAUSES

The majority of cases of acute diarrhea are infectious in origin. Other disorders associated with acute episodes of diarrhea include:

1. Inflammatory bowel disease
2. Neoplastic disease
   a. Intestinal tumors
   b. Extraintestinal tumors, especially carcinoid and pancreatic tumors (Zollinger-Ellison syndrome)
3. Endocrine disorders, especially diabetes and hyperthyroidism
4. Malabsorption syndromes, such as celiac disease, pancreatic insufficiency, and lactose intolerance
5. Drug-induced diarrhea, including laxatives, antacids containing MgOH, digitalis, quinidine, colchicine, ganglionic blocking agents
6. Functional diarrhea, due to nervousness, emotional stress, or physical exhaustion

## DIARRHEA: DIAGNOSTIC APPROACH AND THERAPY

### History

1. Acute vs chronic vs episodic, noting date of onset
2. Description of diarrhea
   a. Frequency of defecation, amount, and relationship to meals
   b. Character of stool
      i. Watery, bloody, fatty, color, odor
      ii. Large stools vs small stools: (a) if consistently large, source of pathology is more likely small bowel or proximal colon; (b) if consistently small, more likely left colon or rectum; (c) when inflammation is widespread, as in most infectious causes, both patterns are likely to be seen
   c. Time of day (functional diarrhea usually occurs only during the day, whereas diarrhea from organic causes may occur both during the day and night)
   d. Associated systemic symptoms: fever, arthritis, arthralgias
3. Background
   a. Foods eaten within last 72 hours
   b. Recent travel
   c. Contact with similarly afflicted persons
   d. Any family or community epidemics
   e. Current medications (especially laxatives, antacids, and antibiotics)
   f. Underlying medical problems (e.g., diabetes, inflammatory bowel disease, hemorrhoids, etc.)
   g. Underlying emotional stress

### Physical Examination

1. Look for evidence of dehydration and systemic involvement
2. Abdominal exam: look for signs of obstruction, peritonitis, organomegaly, masses
3. Rectal exam: digital exam and, if there is bleeding, proctoscopy; look for masses; stool sample for blood

### Tests

1. CBC
2. Serum electrolytes
3. Stool examined for PMNs, blood, mucus, fat, ova, parasites
4. Stool culture and guaiac

These tests will usually suffice, but with severe abdominal pain or grossly bloody stools, other tests may be required, especially:

1. Sigmoidoscopy (with bloody stools)
2. Abdominal x-rays (with severe pain, bloating, or signs of obstruction or peritonitis)
3. Malabsorption workup
4. Rectal biopsy (in patients with inflammatory bowel disease)

## Therapy

Few patients will actually require any intervention. When indicated, however, immediate supportive measures may include:

1. IV fluids
2. Blood transfusion
3. Electrolyte replacement
4. Treatment of the underlying disease when possible

A variety of nonspecific antidiarrheal agents are available. They should not be used routinely, and in some cases (salmonellosis and shigellosis) may prolong excretion of the organism and hence the duration of the illness. The presence of blood and PMNs in the stool and marked fever early in the course of infectious bowel disease should be considered a contraindication to the use of these drugs.

1. Bulk-forming agents, commonly used as laxatives, can also relieve acute diarrhea because of their ability to absorbe water and form an emollient mass.
2. Absorbents: the most popular is Kaopectate
3. Narcotics include:
   a. Paregoric
   b. Codeine
   c. Diphenoxylate (Lomotil contains diphenoxylate plus atropine sulfate); side effects are nausea, vomiting, dizziness and, uncommonly, pruritis and skin rash; use with caution in patients with severe liver disease and severe colitis

## COMMON INFECTIOUS CAUSES
## OF ACUTE DIARRHEA

### Staphylococcal food poisoning

1. Mode of transmission: inadequately cooked meat or improperly refrigerated dairy products
2. Signs and symptoms: nausea, vomiting, no fever; diarrhea can be explosive and voluminous
3. Stool exam: no characteristic findings; PMNs are not present.
4. Treatment: symptomatic
5. Comments: onset 1–6 hours after ingestion, abates within 12 hours, resolves within 72 hours

### Clostridial food poisoning

1. Mode of transmission: usually meat
2. Signs and symptoms: diarrhea and abdominal cramps, no fever, nausea and vomiting are rare
3. Stool exam: no characteristic findings; PMNs are not present.
4. Treatment: symptomatic
5. Comments: 12–24 hour incubation, disease lasts < 24 hours

### Pseudomembranous colitis

1. Mode of transmission: in debilitated patients and patients taking antibiotics, especially clindamycin and lincomycin (also ampicillin, cephalexin)
2. Signs and symptoms: diarrhea, abdominal pain (can be severe), fever, fluid loss (also may be severe)
3. Stool exam: some blood, mucus, PMNs are present
4. Treatment: supportive treatment; discontinue all antibiotics; administer vancomycin
5. Comments: often due to *Clostridium difficile* in patients on antibiotics; sigmoidoscopy reveals exudative plaques or pseudomembranes

### Salmonellosis

1. Mode of transmission: usually foodborne, especially poultry, eggs, dairy; increased risk in patients with gastric surgery
2. Signs and symptoms: diarrhea, abdominal cramps, nausea, vomiting; fever can be high (but white blood count is normal)
3. Stool exam: PMNs are present (but fewer than shigellosis); culture positive >90% in early stages

4. Treatment: symptomatic; antibiotics are contraindicated (unless systemic signs) since they prolong excretion
5. Comments: 8–48 hours incubation, resolves usually in 3–6 days

## Shigellosis

1. Mode of transmission: usually person to person, occasionally via food, milk, water
2. Signs and symptoms: diarrhea, abdominal cramps; tenesmus is characteristic; nausea and vomiting are mild or absent; fever
3. Stool exam: large amounts of PMNs and blood; mucus may be present; culture usually positive
4. Treatment: symptomatic, but 5-day course of ampicillin may shorten duration
5. Comments: 1–2 day incubation, lasts several days; most common in tropical regions (bacterial dysentery)

## Vibriosis

1. Mode of transmission: raw seafood
2. Signs and symptoms: diarrhea, abdominal cramps, nausea, vomiting, headache, fever
3. Stool exam: blood and PMNs may be present
4. Treatment: symptomatic, can give tetracycline if severe
5. Comments: 9–36 hour incubation, lasts 1–3 days; superficial ulcerations may be seen by proctoscopy

## *E. coli*

1. Mode of transmission: seen in travelers, infants, elderly
2. Signs and symptoms: diarrhea; other symptoms usually mild (malaise, cramps, nausea, vomiting); fever mild or absent
3. Stool exam: PMNs sometimes present, no blood
4. Treatment: symptomatic
5. Comments: called "traveler's diarrhea," onset usually 5–15 days after arrival in new region

## Viral gastroenteritis

1. Mode of transmission: winter epidemics, clusters in families and communities
2. Signs and symptoms: viral prodrome (myalgias, malaise, often respiratory symptoms), then nausea, vomiting, diarrhea; fever mild or absent
3. Stool exam: no PMNs, no blood

## COMMON INFECTIOUS CAUSES
## OF ACUTE DIARRHEA *(cont.)*

4. Treatment: symptomatic
5. Comments: diarrhea may linger after other symptoms subside; mistakenly called intestinal flu

### Giardiasis

1. Mode of transmission: acquired during travel (U.S.S.R., Rocky Mountains)
2. Signs and symptoms: watery diarrhea, fever; can be chronic with recurrent diarrhea and malabsorption
3. Stool exam: trophozoites or cysts in >50% of patients (higher yield from duodenal aspirate); no blood, no PMNs
4. Treatment: metronidazole
5. Comments: malabsorption and weight loss are common

### Amebic gastroenteritis

1. Mode of transmission: usually acquired in tropical regions
2. Signs and symptoms: diarrhea, abdominal pain, may persist chronically with anorexia and malaise or rapidly progress to perforation leading to peritonitis, shock and death
3. Stool exam: blood, mucus, no PMNs; trophozoites (containing ingested red blood cells) seen in stool specimen and in rectal mucosal scrapings from areas of ulceration
4. Treatment: metronidazole, often accompanied by diiodohydroxyquine
5. Comments: sigmosdoscopy reveals ulcers often covered by an exudate with intervening normal mucosa

### *Campylobacter enteritis*

1. Mode of transmission: only recently recognized as major cause of diarrhea, with some cases linked to milk and water
2. Signs and symptoms: severe abdominal pain, diarrhea; fever not always present
3. Stool exam: bloody stools, PMNs
4. Treatment: symptomatic; if severe, can give tetracycline or erythromycin
5. Comments: resembles shigellosis, lasts 1–4 days

## CAUSES OF MALABSORPTION

1. Inadequate digestion: postgastrectomy steatorrhea
2. Bile salt deficiency—impaired micelle formation
   a. Impaired synthesis (severe parenchymal or cholestatic liver disease)
   b. Extrahepatic obstruction (most commonly biliary cirrhosis)
   c. Deconjugation due to bacterial overgrowth in the intestine
      i. Due to stasis: blind loops, strictures, abnormal peristalsis (as in diabetic autonomic neuropathy and intestinal scleroderma), and diverticula (often with achlorhydria in the elderly)
      ii. Due to upper GI contamination via an enterocolic fistula: peptic ulcer disease and granulomatous inflammatory bowel disease
   d. Failure of distal ileum to resorb bile salts
      i. Ileal resection
      ii. Granulomatous ileitis (regional enteritis)
3. Exocrine pancreatic insufficiency—inadequate pancreatic lipase
   a. Chronic pancreatitis, usually due to alcohol abuse
   b. Less common causes include pancreatic cancer and cystic fibrosis
4. Intestinal mucosal abnormalities—impaired absorption
   a. Celiac disease
   b. Tropical sprue
   c. Giardiasis
   d. Amyloidosis
   e. Crohn's disease
   f. Lymphoma
5. Intestinal lymphatic obstruction
   a. Whipple's disease
   b. Lymphoma
   c. Intestinal lymphangiectasia
   d. Kalmeier–Degos
6. Cardiovascular abnormalities
   a. Congestive heart failure
   b. Mesenteric vascular insufficiency
7. Lactase deficiency

## CAUSES OF MALABSORPTION *(cont.)*

8. Miscellaneous causes
   a. Gastrectomy
   b. Endocrine disorders
      i. Diabetes
      ii. Hyperthyroidism
      iii. Hypothyroidism
   c. Drugs
      i. Birth control pills
      ii. Colchicine
      iii. Cholestyramine
      iv. Laxatives
      v. Alcohol
      vi. Neomycin

## MALABSORPTION WORKUP

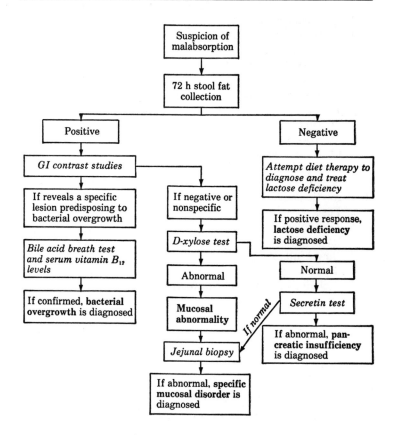

# COMMON CAUSES OF INTESTINAL OBSTRUCTION

1. Mechanical causes
   a. Small bowel
      i. Adhesions
      ii. Neoplasms
      iii. Herniation
      iv. Inflammatory bowel disease
   b. Large bowel
      i. Neoplasms
      ii. Volvulus
      iii. Diverticulitis
      iv. Fecal impaction
      v. Inflammatory bowel disease
2. Paralytic ileus
   a. Postoperative
   b. Peritonitis
   c. Hypokalemia
   d. Bowel infarction
   e. Sepsis
   f. Prolonged mechanical obstruction

## LAXATIVES

### Uses

1. To treat functional constipation on a short-term basis; for long-term relief, a change in diet habits and regular exercise should be encouraged where feasible.
2. To ameliorate pain in anorectal disorders.
3. To ease the passage of stools in patients recovering from a myocardial infarction and in patients who are bedridden, especially postoperatively.
4. To purge the bowel prior to radiologic or endoscopic examination, or before initiation of antihelminthic therapy.
5. To aid in the elimination of some poisons and drugs, e.g., some antihelminthics.

### Side Effects of Excessive Use

1. Crampy abdominal pain.
2. Flatulence.
3. Laxative dependence.
4. Electrolyte disorders, especially dehydration, hypokalemia, alkalosis, hypomagnesemia, and hyponatremia with secondary aldosteronism.
5. Malabsorption syndromes, especially deficiencies of vitamins A, D, E, and K.
6. Cathartic colon (the presence of severe radiologic abnormalities in the colon, commonly seen in women taking laxatives for more than 15 years; of uncertain functional significance).
7. Interference with the absorption of some medications (e.g., laxatives containing cellulose bind digitalis).

### Contraindications

1. Undiagnosed abdominal pain.
2. Intestinal obstruction.
3. Chronic constipation.
4. Gastrointestinal bleeding.
5. Fecal impaction.
6. Allergy (5–7% of population may be allergic to phenolphthalein (Ex-Lax).

## LAXATIVES *(cont.)*

### Types of Laxatives

1. Emollient—surface active wetting agents that permit water and fat to penetrate fecal mass and soften stool; especially useful when straining at stool should be avoided (e.g., in patients post-myocardial infarction or with severe hemorrhoids), [e.g., dioctyl sodium sulfosuccinate (Colace—50-200 mg q.d.) and dioctyl calcium sulfosuccinate (Surfak—240 mg q.d.)].
2. Bulk-forming agents—increase moisture content and mass of stool, thus stimulating reflex peristalsis; gentlest and safest laxatives for prolonged use [e.g., psyllium (Metamucil. 1-2 tbsp. in liquid and methylcellulose (1-5 gm b.i.d.-t.i.d.)].
3. Cathartics—stimulate colon peristalsis; often used to purge the bowel prior to diagnostic studies [e.g., bisacodyl (Dulcolax, 5-10 mg qhs), cascara extracts (4-12 mL qhs), or senna extracts (Senekot, 1 tab qhs)].
4. Saline cathartics—nonabsorbed salts that osmotically retain water in colon lumen; danger of hypermagnesemia in patients with renal failure [e.g. milk of magnesia (15-30 mL qhs) or magnesium titrates (200 mL qhs)].

## CARCINOID SYNDROME: MANIFESTATIONS

This is an uncommon syndrome caused by the release of serotonin, bradykinin, histamine, and other vasoactive substances by malignant tumors usually originating in the GI tract. The full-blown syndrome generally appears only when the tumors have metastasized to the liver. In patients with the less common lung, ovarian, or pericardial carcinoids, liver metastases are not necessary for development of the carcinoid syndrome. Among all patients with carcinoid tumors, only 20% develop the carcinoid syndrome. Diagnosis is made by demonstrating an elevated urinary excretion of 5-hydroxyindoleacetic acid, a metabolite of serotonin.* The clinical course is usually prolonged.

1. Flushing over the face and neck is often precipitated by strong emotions, physical activity, or the ingestion of food or alcohol. An attack of flushing may be accompanied by palpitations, hypotension and abdominal symptoms. Vasomotor disturbances do not include hypertension.
2. GI symptoms include diarrhea, borborygmi, crampy abdominal pain, nausea, and vomiting.
3. Telangiectasias.
4. Fibrosis of pulmonary or tricuspid valves.
5. Increased incidence of peptic ulcer disease.
6. Wheezing, cough, or dysphagia.
7. Arthropathy.
8. Pellagra-like skin lesions.

*A false positive urinary 5-HIAA can result from ingestion of bananas, walnuts, or pineapples, and may also occur in patients with Whipple's disease and celiac disease. False negatives can result from phenothiazine ingestion.

# Section

# 9

# Neurology

## ANALYSIS OF CEREBROSPINAL FLUID

### Method of collection:

1. Measure CSF pressure with manometer; presence of normal respiratory variation insures proper placement of needle.
2. Note opening pressure (normal < 200 mm Hg).
3. Collect four tubes of fluid for analysis:
   a. 1 mL for immediate cell count and analysis
   b. 1–2 mL for culture and lab smears (bacteria, TB, fungi)
   c. 2 mL for glucose and protein
   d. 1–2 mL for lab cell count and serology
4. Note closing pressure
5. Note gross appearance (clear, cloudy, xanthrochromic, bloody)
6. Examine sediment of tube a with:
   a. Gram stain for bacteria
   b. Wright's stain for white blood cell count and differential.
   c. Other stains as indicated (e.g., Ziehl-Neelsen, India ink).
7. Post lumbar puncture care includes bed rest to avoid CSF leakage and resultant headache, and mild analgesics for headache if necessary.

#### Bloody CSF: Intracerebral Hemorrhage vs. Traumatic Tap

| CSF finding | Intracerebral hemorrhage | Traumatic tap |
|---|---|---|
| Xanthrochromia | Yes, if blood present >6 h | No |
| CSF clotting | No | Frequently |
| RBCs in serial tubes | Equal in all tubes | Each successive tube has fewer red blood cells |
| CSF pressure | May be increased | Normal |

## MENINGITIS: CSF PROFILES

| CSF Findings | Normal | Bacterial | Viral (aseptic profile) | Fungal, TB, and partially treated bacterial | Neoplastic |
|---|---|---|---|---|---|
| Leukocyte count | <2 | >500 | <500 | <500 | Usually normal |
| Predominant leukocyte | Lymphocyte | PMN | Lymphocyte | Lymphocyte | Lymphocyte |
| Protein | <50mg/dl | Increased | Normal or slight increase | Normal or slight increase | Increased |
| Glucose | 50–60% of a simultaneous blood glucose | Decreased | Normal | Decreased | Normal or decreased |
| Pressure | 100–200mm | Increased | Normal or increased | Normal or increased | Increased |
| Microscopic exam | — | Gram stain positive in 80% | Negative | Rarely see mycobacteria; India Ink for cryptococcus | Occasionally see neoplastic cells |

Note: The finding of an elevated CSF protein with no other CSF abnormalities, including a normal cell count, may be seen in diabetics, stroke patients, uremics, and chronic alcoholics without meningitis.

## MENINGITIS: PRESENTATION AND ETIOLOGY

### Signs and symptoms

1. Severe headache
2. Fever
3. Stiff neck: related signs of meningeal irritation include Kernig's sign, in which knee extension with the patient sitting elicits pain in the back and hamstrings, and Brudzinski's sign, in which forced neck flexion causes the patient to flex his knees and hips
4. Photophobia
5. Seizures
6. Coma
7. Altered mental status (disorientation, confusion, etc.), which may be the sole finding in an elderly patient

### Major causes

1. Bacterial
   a. *Pneumococcus:* leading cause in adults; sudden onset, frequently presents with seizures or coma
   b. *Meningococcus:* characteristic rash, although an identical rash may be seen with staphylococcus and ECHO virus
   c. *Hemophilus:* leading cause in children
   d. *Listeria:* usually seen in immunosuppressed patients
   e. Gram negative: usually associated with head trauma or following surgery; *Klebsiella, E. coli,* and *Pseudomonas* are the most common
   f. Tuberculosis: usually subacute or chronic; evidence of cranial nerve involvement is common
2. Viral: Patients typically have a viral syndrome prodrome; most run a short and uncomplicated course; the majority of cases are caused by enteroviruses (Coxsackie and ECHO)
3. Fungal
   a. *Cryptococcus:* commonly seen in immunosuppressed patients
   b. *Coccidiodes:* in southwest United States
   c. *Candida*
4. Neoplastic disease
   a. Leukemia
   b. Metastases to CNS
5. Other causes of meningitis, such as sarcoid and SLE, are much less common

## CAUSES OF PAPILLEDEMA*

1. Cranial: increased intracranial pressure
   a. Space-occupying lesions: edema, tumor, brain abscess, bleeding
   b. Meningitis
   c. Pseudotumor cerebri
   d. Leukemia or lymphoma with CNS involvement
2. Orbital and ocular
   a. Tumors (may be unilateral)
   b. Graves' ophthalmopathy
   c. Glaucoma
   d. Uveitis
   e. Injuries
3. Systemic
   a. Hypertension
   b. Hypoventilation with $CO_2$ retention
   c. Uremia
   d. Hypercalcemia
   e. Anemia, acute blood loss
4. Toxic
   a. Methanol
   b. CO poisoning
   c. Lead poisoning

*Gottlieb AJ, et al.: Whole Internist Catalog, p. 117. Philadelphia, WB Saunders, 1980.

## COMA: COMMON CAUSES

### Structural lesions

1. Vascular disease
   a. Intracerebral hemorrhage
   b. Subdural hematoma
   c. Epidural hematoma
   d. Subarachnoid hemorrhage
   e. Cerebral infarction
2. Infection
   a. Meningitis
   b. Encephalitis
   c. Subdural empyema
   d. Brain abscess
3. Tumors
   a. Primary (most commonly gliomas)
   b. Metastases (most commonly from the lungs, breats, GI, kidney)
4. Seizures
5. Status epilepticus
6. Concussion, contusion

### Metabolic causes

1. Drugs and toxins
   a. Alcohol
   b. Carbon monoxide
   c. Heavy metals
   d. Salicylates, opiates, barbiturates, sedatives, tranquilizers, and others
2. Fluid, electrolyte and acid-base disorders: virtually all, if severe enough
3. Hypoxia
   a. All causes of decreased cardiac output
   b. Anemia
   c. Respiratory failure
   d. Hypo- and hypertension

4. Endocrine disease
   a. Diabetes mellitus
   b. Hypoglycemia
   c. Hypo- and hyperthyroidism
   d. Hypo- and hyperpituitarism
   e. Hypo- and hyperadrenalism
   f. Hypo- and hyperparathyroidism
5. Hepatic encephalopathy
6. Uremia
7. Heat stroke and hypothermia
8. Vitamin deficiencies (e.g., thiamine deficiency leading to Wernicke's encephalopathy)
9. Systemic diseases (e.g., SLE, SBE)

## PROGRESSION OF NEUROLOGIC CHANGES IN COMA

With increasing damage to the central nervous system, a characteristic pattern of neurologic changes can frequently be observed.

### Respirations

1. Cheyne–Stokes breathing (periods of rapid breathing alternating with periods of apnea) signifies either damage to the cerebral hemispheres or metabolic encephalopathy.
2. Central hyperventilation, sustained hyperpnea, signifies damage to the lower midbrain and upper pons.
3. Apneustic breathing, typified by extended pauses in inspiration, signifies damage to the lower pons.
4. Chaotic breathing, totally without any regularity, signifies medullary involvement.

### Pupillary responses

1. Metabolic causes of coma produce no pattern of altered responses, although certain drugs may give large or small pupils.
2. With structural lesions, the pupils become fixed at mid position with midbrain damage.
3. Pontine damage leaves the pupils small or pinpoint.

### Extraocular movements

1. Paralysis of extraocular movements in the doll's eyes maneuver* indicates midbrain and pontine damage.

*Doll's eyes can only be demonstrated in patients who are comatose with intact midbrain and pontine function.

## COMA: IMMEDIATE MANAGEMENT

1. Assure adequacy of ventilation and circulation.
2. Control body temperature.
3. Establish IV line.
4. Obtain blood and urine samples.
5. Deliver
   a. IV glucose (50 mL of 50% solution)
   b. IV naloxone (Narcan) (0.4–0.8 mg)
6. Treat seizures.
7. Correct fluid, electrolyte, acid-base imbalances.
8. Treat infection.
9. CT scan is now the method of choice for diagnosing intracranial lesions, and should precede an LP if a mass lesion is suspected.

## SYNCOPE: DIFFERENTIAL DIAGNOSIS

1. Neurogenic (vasovagal syncope): strong emotion or pain induces a sudden hypotensive epidose; perhaps the most common cause of fainting
2. Orthostatic hypotension
   a. Drugs (antihypertensive medications, MAO inhibitors, tricyclic antidepressants, phenothiazines, barbiturates, vincristine, L-dopa, quinidine)
   b. Hypovolemia (often secondary to diuretics or blood loss)
   c. Neurologic deficits (seen in diabetes, tabes dorsalis, pernicious anemia, Parkinson's disease)
   d. Shy–Drager syndrome
   e. Idiopathic
3. Cardiac disease (via low output because of pump failure, outflow obstruction, or arrhythmia)
   a. Arrhythmias (both brady- and tachyarrhythmias, frequently in a setting of ischemia or infarction)
   b. Heart block
      i. AV block (Stokes–Adams attacks)
      ii. Sinoatrial block (sick sinus syndrome)
   c. Asymmetric septal hypertrophy (ASH)
   d. Aortic stenosis
   e. Atrial myxoma
   f. Mitral valve prolapse
   g. Cardiac tamponade
4. Less common causes
   a. Carotid sinus syndrome
   b. Cerebrovascular disease
   c. Hysterical syncope (usually in young women)
   d. Hypoglycemia
   e. Anemia
   f. Hyperventilation
   g. Micturition syncope (usually in elderly men)
   h. Glossopharyngeal neuralgia

## MUSCLE WEAKNESS: LOCATING THE LESION

### Central nervous system

1. Weakness is lateralized and focal.
2. Early atrophy is not prominent.
3. Deep tendon reflexes are increased and muscle tone is spastic (although acutely muscle tone is flaccid).
4. Pathologic reflexes (e.g., Babinski) may be present.
5. Common causes: infarction, hemorrhage, tumors.

### Anterior horn cells

1. Weakness is scattered.
2. Early atrophy is prominent.
3. Fasciculations can be seen.
4. No sensory abnormalities (unlike Guillain-Barre).
5. In amyotropic lateral sclerosis (ALS), upper neurons are also involved and thus there is spasticity, increased tendon reflexes, and pathologic reflexes. In poliomyelitis, reflexes are diminished and muscle tone is flaccid.
6. Causes: amyotropic lateral sclerosis and poliomyelitis.

### Peripheral nerves and nerve roots

1. Weakness is predominantly distal.
2. Atrophy may be profound.
3. Deep tendon reflexes are decreased and muscle tone is flaccid.
4. Fasciculations can be seen, and EMG shows fibrillations.
5. Sensory abnormalities confirm neurogenic rather than myogenic origin.
6. Common causes: neuropathies (e.g., diabetic), inflammation, disc herniation, Guillain-Barre syndrome.

### Neuromuscular junction

1. Weakness is generally proximal, improves with anticholinesterase administration.
2. Prominent symptom is easy fatigability.
3. EMG reveals diminishing response to repeated stimuli.
4. Common cause: myasthenia gravis.

## MUSCLE WEAKNESS: LOCATING THE LESION *(cont.)*

### Skeletal muscle

1. Weakness tends to be more proximal.
2. Atrophy appears late in disease course.
3. Deep tendon reflexes are usually normal.
4. No sensory abnormalities.
5. Muscles are tender in polymyositis.
6. EMG reveals brief, low voltage potentials.
7. Common causes: polymyositis, myotonia, muscular distrophy.

## TREMORS*

| | Resting (static) tremor | Postural (action) tremor | Intention (ataxic) tremor |
|---|---|---|---|
| Descrip- | Occurs while patient is at rest | Appears during attempt to maintain a posture | Appears only during precise coordinated movement |
| Test | Observe patient at rest | Observe patient standing with arms overhead, hands extended | Observe fine movements: finger to nose and heel to shin |
| Etiology | Parkinson's disease | Benign essential tremor,† cerebellar disease, hyperthyroidism, anxiety, fatigue, drug withdrawal, alcoholism, mercury poisoning, pheochromocytoma, liver failure (asterixis), uremia, $CO_2$ narcosis | Cerebellar disease, multiple sclerosis, phenytoin toxicity |

*Wilson's disease can present with any of the three types of tremor.
†Benign essential tremor is frequently reduced by alcohol.

## VERTIGO

### Differential Diagnosis

1. Vestibular diseases
   a. Benign positional vertigo
   b. Meniere's disease
   c. Middle ear infections
   d. Vestibular neuronitis
   e. Allergic labyrinthitis
   f. Ototoxic drugs (especially the aminoglycoside antibiotics)
2. Central disorders
   a. Acoustic neuromas (and less common tumors of the cerebello-pontine angle)
   b. Vertebrobasilar insufficiency
   c. Multiple sclerosis
   d. Epilepsy
   e. Cerebrovascular accident
   f. Subclavian steal syndrome
   g. Postconcussion
   h. Metabolic diseases
3. Other causes
   a. Psychiatric (hyperventilation, anxiety, etc.)
   b. Volume depletion
   c. Anemia
   d. Syncope
   e. Hypothyroidism

### Peripheral vs. Central Lesions

|  | *Peripheral (vestibular)* | *Central* |
|---|---|---|
| Nystagmus | Latency before onset; transient (<1 min) | No latency; persistent (>1 min); verticle nystagmus implies a branstem lesion |
| Calorics | Decreased on side of lesion (normal in benign positional nystagmus) | Normal (decreased in acoustic neuroma) |
| Description of vertigo | Severe, often rotational | Mild |
| Nausea, vomiting | Usually present | Usually absent |
| Hearing loss, tinnitus | Frequently present | Absent (loss of high tones in acoustic neuroma) |

## A Simple Classification

1. Generalized
   a. Grand mal
   b. Petit mal
   c. Other (e.g., akinetic, myoclonic)

2. Focal
   a. Simple motor (e.g., Jacksonian)
   b. Simple sensory
   c. Temporal lobe (psychomotor or complex partial)

|  | *Grand mal* | *Petit mal* | *Temporal lobe* |
|---|---|---|---|
| Description | Heralded by aura; sudden loss of consciousness followed by tonic, then clonic muscle contractions of head and limbs; fecal and urinary incontinence are frequent; attack lasts several minutes, followed by postictal disorientation | Sudden loss of awareness ("absence") lasts at most 30 seconds and may occur many times during each day | May be an aura, usually a sensory illusion or hallucination; patient then loses contact with environment and engages in automatic activity— moving about, trying to speak, etc.; will not respond to questions and may become violent if restrained; attack usually lasts several minutes |

*(continued)*

## SEIZURES (cont.)

| | Grand mal | Petit mal | Temporal lobe |
|---|---|---|---|
| Age of onset | Any age | 4–8 years | Usually 10–30 years |
| EEG | 25–30/s high voltage spikes over any area of cortex | 3/s spike and wave (generalized) | Spike or slow wave focus over one temporal lobe |
| First line drugs | Phenytoin (Dilantin) | Ethosuximide (Zarontin) | Phenytoin |
| | Phenobarbitol | Acetazolamide (Diamox) | Primidone (Mysoline) |
| | Primidone | Clonazepam (Clonopin) | Carbamazepine (Tegretol) |
| | Carbamazepine | Trimethadione | Frequently requires a combination of drugs |

# SIDE EFFECTS OF SOME COMMON ANTICONVULSANTS

1. Phenobarbital (Luminal)*
   a. Half-life: 120 hours
   b. Side effects: sedation, nystagmus, ataxia, skin rash, megaloblastic anemia, osteomalacia
2. Phenytoin (Dilantin)†
   a. Half-life: 24 hours.
   b. Side effects: nystagmus, ataxia, GI upset, skin rash, gingival hypertrophy, hirsutism, pseudolymphoma, blood dyscrasias, SLE-like syndrome, dysarthria, osteomalacia
3. Primidone (Mysoline)‡
   a. Half-life: 12 hours
   b. Side effects: sedation, vertigo, nausea, vomiting, allergic rash, megaloblastic anemia, ataxia, SLE-like syndrome, impotence, pitting edema, personality changes
4. Carbamazepine (Tegretol)
   a. Half-life: 12 hours
   b. Side effects: sedation, dizziness, diplopia, nystagmus, skin rash, GI upset, jaundice, blood dyscrasias, dry mouth, ataxia
   c. Teratogenic.
5. Ethosuximide (Zarontin)
   a. Half-life: 48–72 hours
   b. Side effects: sedation, ataxia, GI upset, fatigue, lethargy, headache, dizziness, grand mal seizures, pancytopenia, SLE-like syndrome, skin rash
6. Acetazolamide (Diamox)
   a. Half-life: 6–12 hours
   b. Side effects: hyperchloremic acidosis, GI upset, nephrolithiasis
7. Clonazepam (Clonopin)
   a. Half-life: 24–32 hours
   b. Side effects: sedation
8. Trimethadione (Tridrone)
   a. Half-life: 12–24 hours
   b. Side effects: sedation, photophobia, diplopia, headache, vertigo, blood dyscrasias, nephrotic syndrome, grand mal seizures, dermatitis, hepatitis

*Overdose can cause fatal respiratory depression; withdrawal seizures respond only to high-dose barbiturates.
†Not sedative; overdose is not fatal; withdrawal seizures do not occur.
‡Effects of overdose and withdrawal are similar to phenobarbital.

## THE MAJOR STROKE SYNDROMES
## DESCRIBED BY LOCATION

A stroke may result from thrombosis, embolism, or hemorrhage of
a cerebral artery. The resulting neurologic manifestations depend
upon the particular artery that is affected. The following list includes
findings that may occur when a given artery is occluded.

1. Middle cerebral artery
    a. Contralateral hemiplegia (may be severe)
    b. Contralateral hemianesthesia
    c. Homonymous hemianopia
    d. Paresis of conjugate gaze to opposite side
    e. Aphasia (if dominant hemisphere), apraxia or anosognosia
       (if nondominant hemisphere)
2. Anterior cerebral artery
    a. contralateral hemiplegia (or paresis), usually affecting the leg
       and foot
    b. Urinary incontinence
    c. Infantile reflexes
    d. Contralateral hemianesthesia, also usually affecting the leg
       and foot
    e. Behavioral and emotional changes (e.g., abulia, euphoria)
    f. Gaze apraxia
3. Internal carotid artery: any of the manifestrations of (1) and (2)
   plus transient monocular blindness
4. Posterior cerebral artery
    a. Homonymous hemianopia (may be upper quadrantic)
    b. Contralateral hemianesthesia
    c. Memory loss
    d. Dyslexia
    e. Contralateral involuntary movements (typically hemiballis-
       mus)
5. Vertebrobasilar artery
    a. Ipsilateral cranial nerve abnormalities
    b. Contralateral motor and sensory abnormalities
    c. Nausea, vomiting
    d. Vertigo
    e. Ataxia
    f. Dystharthria
    g. Emotional lability

## FEATURES OF STROKE SYNDROMES DESCRIBED BY ETIOLOGY

| | Embolus | Intracerebral bleed | Thrombosis | Lacunar state | Subarachnoid hemorrhage |
|---|---|---|---|---|---|
| Site | Peripheral | Deep | Variable | Pons, internal capsule, basal ganglia | Variable |
| Onset | Sudden with maximal deficit at onset | Sudden with development of signs over minutes to hours | Gradual with stepwise or stuttering onset over hours to days | Gradual with stepwise or stuttering onset | Sudden |
| Context | Active | Active | Inactive | Inactive | Active |
| TIAs? | None | None | Usually | Occasionally | None |
| LP | Usually clear | Usually bloody | Clear | Clear | Bloody |
| Headache | Yes | Yes | Yes | No | Yes |

After Werner HL, Levitt LP: Neurology for the house officer. Baltimore: Williams & Wilkins, 1974, pp 21–22. © (1974) The Williams & Wilkins Co., Baltimore.

## MULTIPLE SCLEROSIS:
## THE MOST COMMON SIGNS AND SYMPTOMS

1. Weakness
2. Spasticity and pathologic reflexes
3. Impaired vision
4. Impaired sensation (most commonly vibration and position sense)
5. Vertigo
6. Autonomic impairment: bladder, bowel, and sexual dysfunction
7. Cerebellar signs: intention tremor and ataxia
8. Mood alterations: emotional lability, depression, euphoria
9. Loss of medial gaze during conjugate eye movements, but able to converge

## CAUSES OF HEADACHE

1. Psychogenic
   a. Tension headache
   b. Neurotic headache
2. Vascular
   a. Migraine
   b. Cluster headache
   c. Hypertensive headache
   d. Temporal arteritis
3. Intracranial
   a. Brain tumor and other expanding lesions (brain abscess, subdural hematoma)
   b. Subarachnoid hemorrhage
   c. Meningitis and encephalitis
   d. Lumbar puncture headache
4. Extracranial
   a. Sinusitis
   b. Lesions of the eye, ear, oral cavity, and cervical spine
5. Miscellaneous
   a. Neural dysfunction (e.g., trigeminal neuralgia)
   b. Posttraumatic headache
   c. Associated with systemic illness (fever, infection, hypoglycemia, etc.)

The following lists describe several of the more common varieties of headache.

1. *Psychogenic: tension headache*
   a. Location—bilateral, base of skull, may radiate to front and be described as a bandlike constriction around the head
   b. Duration—usually hours, sometimes days, rarely weeks or longer
   c. Description—steady, nonpulsatile aching, tightness, or pressure; no systemic or neurologic findings; head and neck muscles may be tender
   d. Mechanism—excessive sustained muscle contractions of head and neck almost always related to anxiety or other emotional stress
   e. Therapy—generally responds to aspirin or acetaminophin; if frequent, a tranquilizer (such as diazepam) may help; heat or massage may help mild headaches

## CAUSES OF HEADACHE *(cont.)*

   f. Comments—a variant, the neurotic headache, is usually related to severe underlying depression or anxiety, and persists relentlessly for days, weeks or longer. Antidepressants and psychotherapy may be required

2. *Vascular: cluster headaches*
   a. Location—unilateral, generally in or behind one eye
   b. Duration—minutes to hours
   c. Description—very severe (often described as "stabbing"), abrupt onset, occurs repetitively for days or weeks, frequently at the same time of day; will awaken patient from sleep; accompanied by tears, redness, rhinorrhea, flushing and sweating on affected side of face (an ipsilateral Horner's syndrome may be present, although other autonomic manifestations are rare); may be several attacks per day or only two or three a week during a cluster; remissions between clusters can last weeks, months or years
   d. Mechanism—alcohol is the only known precipitant; the cause of most attacks is unknown; blood histamine levels are elevated; unlike migraines, serotonin levels do not fall
   e. Therapy—ergotamine, methysergide and corticosteroids may be helpful
   f. Comments—more common in men; no family history; attacks are shorter than migraines and more frequent; without an aura

3. *Vascular: migraine*
   a. Location—usually unilateral in patients with classic migraine, otherwise may be bilateral; can affect any area of the head or neck
   b. Duration—hours to days
   c. Description—headache is throbbing, may be mild or—more often—severe; autonomic symptoms include nausea, vomiting, diarrhea, oliguria or diuresis, sweating, pallor, etc.; dizziness, vertigo, or syncope may be present; photophobia and sensitivity to loud noises are common; weakness and fatigue may occur; attack is often followed by a tension headache. Patients with classic migraine (~15%) have a preceding aura, usually visual (flashing or zigzag lights, blind spots, geometric patterns), but may be sensory, motor, or aural (spoken words)
   d. Mechanism—intracranial vasoconstriction followed by extracranial vasodilatation; vasoactive substances (e.g., serotonin) may be involved; many potential triggers: stress, alcohol, tyramine-containing foods (cheese, chocolate), birth control pills, menstruation

e. Therapy—Treat acute attack with ergot alkaloids (often in combination with caffeine or phenobarbitol) at first sign of headache; prophylaxis with methysergide (a serotonin antagonist) or propranolol

f. Comments—>50% have a positive family history; more common in women; usually commences before age 20; rare forms of migraine include hemiplegic migraine (slowly resolving neurologic defects), ophthalmoplegic migraine, and basilar migraine (brain stem involvement)

4. *Vascular: hypertension*

a. Location: frequently diffuse, occasionally most severe over occiput

b. Duration—weeks

c. Description—severe throbbing headache, often worse in the morning

d. Mechanism—generally seen only in patients whose diastolic blood pressure exceeds 120 mm Hg or whose systolic blood pressure exceeds 200 mm Hg (approximately 10% of those patients experience headaches); poorly correlated with fluctuating blood pressure

e. Therapy—treat hypertension, can attempt symptomatic relief with analgesics

f. Comments—may presage an incipient CVA

5. *Vascular: temporal arteritis*

a. Location—temporal regions, often unilateral

b. Duration—weeks

c. Description—throbbing headache, often with systemic signs of fever, malaise, myalgia, weight loss; ESR is elevated, usually >50 mm/hr; temporal arteries are swollen and tender (biopsy confirms diagnosis); often associated with inflammation of intracranial vessels as well, and is a major cause of blindness in the elderly; 50% of affected patients have some type of visual disturbance

d. Mechanism—inflammation of the temporal arteries

e. Therapy—corticosteroids; therapy must be prompt to avert the possibility of blindness or stroke

f. Comments—most often seen in elderly women

6. *Intracranial: brain tumors and mass lesions*

a. Location—often diffuse, especially with elevated intracranial pressure; approximately one third overlie or are near the site of the tumor

b. Duration—may last only minutes or be continuous

## CAUSES OF HEADACHE *(cont.)*

   c. Description—steady, dull, nonthrobbing headache that worsens with cough, changing position, exertion: often worse on awakening after recumbence; may be accompanied by nausea, vomiting (may be projectile), seizures, focal neurologic deficits, other signs and symptoms of an intracranial mass lesion; suspicion should be heightened by the onset of a new headache pattern that progressively worsens

   d. Mechanism—either local irritation of pain-sensitive structures or mass displacement of these structures

   e. Therapy—treatment of the tumor; aspirin may ameliorate the pain

   f. Comments—a similar picture can occur with the syndrome of pseudotumor cerebri (headache, visual deterioration)

7. *Intracranial: subarachnoid hemorrhage*

   a. Location—usually frontal or diffuse, often radiating to the neck

   b. Duration—hours to days

   c. Description—acute onset, very severe and constant, often followed swiftly by mental confusion; meningeal signs may be present and lumbar puncture may reveal blood; nausea, vomiting, lethargy and focal neurologic signs may be seen

   d. mechanism—head trauma, spontaneous rupture of an aneurysm, or a blood dyscrasia are the common causes of subarachnoid hemorrhage, which then damages tissues and induces vascular spasm

   e. Therapy—stabilize the patient, then treat the underlying disorder

8. *Intracranial: meningitis*

   a. Location—usually diffuse, although worse occipitally and frequently radiating down the neck

   b. Duration—days

   c. Description—severe throbbing headache with meningeal signs; lumbar puncture reveals one of several CSF profiles; malaise, fever and vomiting are typical; lethargy, irritability, confusion and seizures may develop

   d. mechanism—lowered pain threshold of inflamed tissues, especially at the base of the brain

   e. Therapy—treat infection where possible

   f. Comments—a similar picture can be seen with encephalitis

9. *Sinusitis*
   a. Location—facial pain over the regions of the frontal and maxillary sinuses
   b. Duration—hours
   c. Description—dull, aching, headache that is very position sensitive; usually begins early in the day and subsides in the evening; nausea and vomiting are rare; rhinorrhea and fever may be seen
   d. Mechanism—mucosal inflammation
   e. Therapy—decongestants and analgesics

# Section

# 10

# Miscellaneous Lists

## COMMON REASONS FOR ANTIBIOTIC FAILURE*

1. Human factors
   a. Incorrect diagnosis
   b. Incorrect medicine given
   c. Failure of patient compliance
   d. Contaminated intravenous lines
2. Drug factors
   a. Inadequate dose
   b. Intervals between doses are too long
   c. Improper route of administration
   d. Incompatibility of drugs mixed in intravenous fluids
   e. Interference by another drug with gastrointestinal absorption
   f. Inadequate penetration of drug to site of infection
   g. Drug fever
3. Pathogen factors
   a. Drug resistance
   b. Superinfection
   c. Infection is in a dormant phase
4. Host factors
   a. Failure to drain, debride, or remove foreign body or other obstruction where necessary
   b. Phlebitis at intravenous site or abscess at intramuscular site
   c. Coexisting serious illness
   d. Depression of immunologic defenses
   e. Normal variation in the expected clinical course

*Adapted from Gardner, P: Hosp Prac 11:41, 1976.

## FEVER OF UNKNOWN ORIGIN (FUO)

The causes of persistent, undiagnosed fever fall into four general categories, listed here in order of decreasing frequency:

1. Infectious diseases
2. Neoplastic diseases
3. Connective tissue diseases
4. Miscellaneous diseases

As many as 20% of cases are never successfully diagnosed. Within each category, certain disease entities figure most often in the ultimate diagnosis. Their incidence varies widely among different series. The most frequent diagnoses are listed below, roughly in order of decreasing frequency:

### Common Causes of FUO of More Than Three Weeks Duration

1. *Infection*
    a. Tuberculosis
    b. Urinary tract infections
    c. Infectious endocarditis
    d. Osteomyelitis
    e. Localized abscesses (most often intraabdominal)
    f. Biliary infections
    g. Fungi and unusual pathogens
2. *Neoplasia*
    a. Hematologic/immunologic malignancies (including Hodgkin's disease, non-Hodgkin's lymphomas, leukemia, and pre-leukemia)
    b. Solid tumors (especially hypernephroma, hepatoma, GI carcinoma, and atrial myxomas)
    c. Widely disseminated cancer
3. *Connective tissue diseases*
    a. Vasculitis [most often giant cell (temporal) arteritis]
    b. SLE
    c. Rheumatoid arthritis
    d. Polyarteritis nodosa
    e. Rheumatic fever
4. *Miscellaneous Diseases*
    a. Juvenile rheumatoid arthritis
    b. Granulomatous diseases (especially sarcoidosis and granulomatous hepatitis)

## FEVER OF UNKNOWN ORIGIN (FUO) *(cont.)*

    c. Factitious fever
    d. Drug reaction
    e. Pulmonary embolus
    f. Inflammatory bowel disease
    g. Alcoholic hepatitis
    h. Thyroiditis
    i. Whipple's disease
    j. Familial Mediterranean fever

### Notes

1. Any solid tumor can cause fever by obstruction leading to infection. Those tumors listed above can cause fever without secondary infection.
2. As the duration of fever increases, the likelihood that infection is responsible decreases.
3. In FUO of greater than 6 months, the following are the most likely diagnoses (in order of decreasing frequency):
    a. Factitious fever
    b. Granulomatous diseases
    c. Neoplastic diseases
    d. Juvenile rheumatoid arthritis
    e. Infection
    f. Connective tissue diseases

## DRUG FEVER*

Any drug can cause fever in a hypersensitive individual. The following list includes those drugs most often implicated in FUO, often without any other signs or symptoms of drug hypersensitivity.

1. Antihistamines
2. Barbiturates
3. Chlorambucil
4. Dilantin
5. Hydralazine
6. Ibuprofen
7. Iodides
8. Isoniazid
9. Mercaptopurine
10. Methyldopa
11. Nitrofurantoin
12. Para-aminosalicylic acid
13. Penicillins
14. Procainamide
15. Quinidine
16. Salicylates
17. Thiouracil

*From Mandell, Douglas, Bennett: Principles and practice of infectious diseases. New York: Wiley, 1979, p. 415. Reprinted with permission of John Wiley & Sons, Inc.

## BURNS*

| Classification of burns | Surface appearance | Sensation | Outcome/ prognosis |
| --- | --- | --- | --- |
| First-degree | Dry, erythematous, no blisters | Painful, hypersensitive | Complete healing within 1 week; no scar |
| Second-degree (superficial) | Blisters, red oozing base, good capillary refill, blanching on pressure | Painful, extremely sensitive to pinprick | Complete healing within 3 weeks; may be erythematous early after healing |
| Second-degree (deep) | Blisters may be present; pale, indurated areas; | Some insensitive areas; many areas anesthetic to pinprick | Firm, thick scar with loss of hair follicles, sweat glands, and skin pigmentation; healing may take 1 month or more. |
| Third-degree | Pearly white or brown or opaque gray; firm, leathery, dry | No sensation | Total skin loss includes all appendages; heals by scar formation if small |

*From TB Fitzpatrick et al: Dermatology in general medicine, 2nd ed. New York: McGraw-Hill, p. 932. Copyright © (1979). Used with the permission of the McGraw-Hill Book Company.

## CONDITIONS ASSOCIATED WITH
## GENERALIZED PRURITUS

1. Uremia: pruritis does not correlate with level of BUN; some experience relief, others worsening with dialysis
2. Jaundice
3. Gout
4. Endocrine disorders
   a. Diabetes mellitus: pruritis may appear early; not related to severity of disease
   b. Hypothyroidism: rarely, hyperthyroidism
   c. Carcinoid syndrome
   d. Hyperparathyroidism
5. Malignancies
   a. Hodgkin's disease
   b. Lymphoma
   c. Leukemia
   d. Mycosis fungoides
   e. Multiple myeloma
   f. Polycythemia: pruritis worse after hot bath or shower
   g. Visceral malignancies very rare
6. Iron deficiency
7. Parasites
   a. hookworm
   b. pinworm
   c. scabies
8. Drug reactions: especially opium derivatives
9. Normal pregnancy: pruritis correlates with serum bilirubin levels
10. Miscellaneous
    a. Dry skin: e.g., winter pruritis
    b. Senile pruritis: itching in the elderly without obvious dry skin
    c. Psychogenic: common!!

## IMPORTANT CAUSES OF GENERALIZED
## HYPERPIGMENTATION

1. Due to hypermelanosis*
   a. Addison's disease
   b. Hemochromatosis
   c. Diseases affecting the liver
      i. Wilson's disease
      ii. Porphyria cutanea tarda
      iii. Primary biliary cirrhosis
   d. Severe cachexia due to starvation, malabsorption, chronic illness
   e. Vitamin $B_{12}$ or folate deficiency
   f. Pregnancy and oral contraceptives
   g. Scleroderma
   h. Pituitary adenomas secreting MSH
   i. Acromegaly
   j. Drugs
      i. Busulfan and other antineoplastic agents
      ii. Chlorpromazine
      iii. Antimalarials (quinacrine, chloroquine)
      iv. Long-term use of antipsychotic drugs with prolonged exposure to sunlight
2. Due to deposition of metals and chemicals
   a. Arsenic
   b. Bismuth
   c. Silver (argyria)
   d. Gold (chrysiasis)
   e. Mercury

*Hypermelanosis in the epidermis appears brown. In the dermis it appears blue-gray. Generalized hyperpigmentation can be best seen in the palmar creases, body folds, recent scars, and sun-exposed areas.

# CONDITIONS ASSOCIATED WITH NAIL DISORDERS

1. Onycholyis (loosening of the nails)
   a. Thyroid disease (Plummer's nails)
2. Koilonychia (spoon nails)
   a. Iron deficiency anemia
   b. Some normals
3. Longitudinal ridging: hypoparathyroidism
4. Brittleness, splitting and ridging
   a. Raynaud's disease
   b. Scleroderma (rarely severe)
5. Pitting
   a. Psoriasis
   b. Reiter's disease
   c. Rheumatoid arthritis
6. Clubbing: see "Clubbing" list
7. Splinter hemorrhages
   a. Infectious endocarditis
   b. Vasculitis
   c. Trauma
8. Periungual telangiectasias
   a. SLE
   b. Scleroderma
   c. Dermatomyositis
   d. Some normals
9. Changes in pigmentation
   a. White nails
      i. Cirrhosis (Terry's nails; proximally or entirely white)
      ii. Hypoalbuminemia (Muehrcke's lines; parallel white bands)
      iii. Renal failure (half-and-half nails; proximal half is white)
      iv. Arsenic poisoning (Mee's lines; white lines)
   b. Yellow nails: chronic edema
   c. Black nails: Vitamin $B_{12}$ deficiency
      i. Pinta
      ii. Peutz-Jeghers syndrome
   d. Blue-brown nails: antimalarials
   e. Blue lunulae: Wilson's disease
      i. Argyria (nail may be slate gray)

## DIALYZABLE POISONS*

Barbiturates
  Barbital
  Phenobarbital
  Amobarbital
  Pentobarbital
  Butabarbital
  Secobarbital
  Cyclobarbital
  Glutethimide†
Depressants,
    sedatives and
    tranquilizers
  Diphenylhydantoin
  Primidone
  Meprobamate
  Ethchlorvynol†
  Ethinamate
  Ethprylon
  Diphenhydramine
  Methaqualone
  Heroin
  Gallamine triethi-
    odide
  Paraldehyde
  Chloral·hydrate
  Chlordiazepoxide
Antidepressants
  Amphetamine
  Methamphetamine
  Tricyclic secondary
    amines
  Monoamine oxidase
    inhibitors
  Tranylcypromine
  Pargyline
  Phenelzine
  Isocarbonazid
Alcohols
  Ethanol†
  Methanol†
  Isopropanol
  Ethylene glycol

Analgesics
  Acetylsalicylic
    acid
  Methylsalicylate†
  Acetophenetidin
  Dextropropoxy-
    phene
  Paracetamol
Antibiotics
  Streptomycin
  Kanamycin
  Neomycin
  Vancomycin
  Penicillin
  Ampicillin
  Sulfonamides
  Cephalin
  Chloramphenicol
  Tetracycline
  Nitrofurantoin
  Polymyxin
  Isoniazid
  Cycloserine
  Quinine
Metals
  Arsenic
  Copper
  Calcium
  Iron
  Lead
  Lithium
  Magnesium
  Mercury
  Potassium
  Sodium
  Strontium
Halides
  Bromide†
  Chloride†
  Iodide
  Fluoride

Endogenous
    toxins
  Ammonia
  Uric acid†
  Tritium†
  Bilirubin
  Lactic acid
  Schizophrenia
  Myasthenia gravis
  Porphyria
  Cystine
  Endotoxin
  Hyperosmolar
    state†
  Water intoxication
Miscellaneous
    substances
  Thiocyanate†
  Aniline
  Sodium chlorate
  Potassim chlorate
  Eucalyptus oil
  Boric acid
  Potassium
    dichromate
  Chromic acid
  Digoxin
  Sodium citrate
  Dinitroorthocresol
  Amanita phalloides
  Carbon tetra-
    chloride
  Ergotamine
  Cyclophosphamide
  5-Fluorouracil
  Methotrexate
  Camphor
  Trichlorethylene
  Carbon monoxide
  Chlorpropamide

*Schreiner GE: Transactions of the American Society for Artificial Organs, 1970.

†Kinetics of dialysis thoroughly studied and/or clinical experience extensive.